"When two souls—the parent's and the child's—both collaborate to bring out the most magnificent qualities within the child, then magic happens, and the world is changed forever. This book provides mothers and fathers with an inspired and practical blueprint for conscious spiritual parenting. Sweetness, serenity and joy shine from its pages, as well as powerful techniques for healing the wounds left by old family patterns."

—Neale Donald Walsch
Author of the *Conversations With God* series

Communing With the Spirit of Your Unborn Child

A Practical Guide to Intimate Communication With Your Unborn or Infant Child

Dawson Church
www.Communing.com

Elite Books
Author's Publishing Cooperative
Santa Rosa, CA 95403
www.Elitebooks.biz

Library of Congress Cataloging-in-Publication Data:

Church, Dawson, 1956-
    **Communing with the spirit of your unborn child : a practical
guide to intimate communication with your unborn or infant
child / Dawson Church. -- 2nd ed.**
    p. cm.
    ISBN 0-9720028-1-2

    1. Pregnancy. 2. Bioenergetics. 3. Breathing exercises. 4. Parent and
child. I. Title
RG525.C63 2004
618.2'4--dc22

2004013815

Cover and Interior design by Authors Publishing Cooperative
Photographs at chapter starts courtesy of Rubberball Productions
(www.rubberball.com)
All other photographs courtesy of Michael B. Buchanan
(www.MichaelBPhotography.com)
Typeset in Colonna and Hoeffler Text
Printed in USA
Second Edition

10 9 8 7 6 5 4 3 2 1

CONTENTS

EXERCISES

Dedication

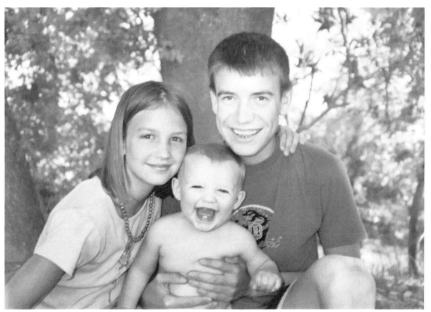

This book is dedicated to my three children, Lionel, Angela & Alexander.
And also to the many women of vision and courage
I have been fortunate to meet. Their wisdom, compassion and insight
have shaped my life.

ACKNOWLEDGMENTS

Much appreciation to the many people who contributed to this book. Thanks to my father, a man amongst men, who has long modeled integrity, consistency and vision in the midst of the trials of life. Thanks to my former wife Brenda, who practiced these techniques with me during the gestation of our children. Special thanks to the many mothers and fathers who told me their stories of communing with their unborn children, and helped me to understand that my experience is not uncommon. Thanks to my teachers in the classes in which I learned these simple yet remarkably effective techniques (www.SoulHealings.com).

Thanks too to the parents who wrote to me or called me to tell me what a difference this book made in their lives, and to Aslan Publishing's Barbara Levine; the encouragement they all gave me to write a new edition of this book contributed to my eventually doing so.

Thanks also to the many friends who buoy me in an unshakable network of support and encouragement, and to the mentors and role models of enlightened living who have inspired me from the earliest times, especially those who have contributed their wisdom to my anthologies, or lent their kind words of endorsement to this book.

Thanks most of all to the Great Spirit who daily nourishes me and fills me with the delight of living.

PART ONE

*Parenting as a
Soul Journey*

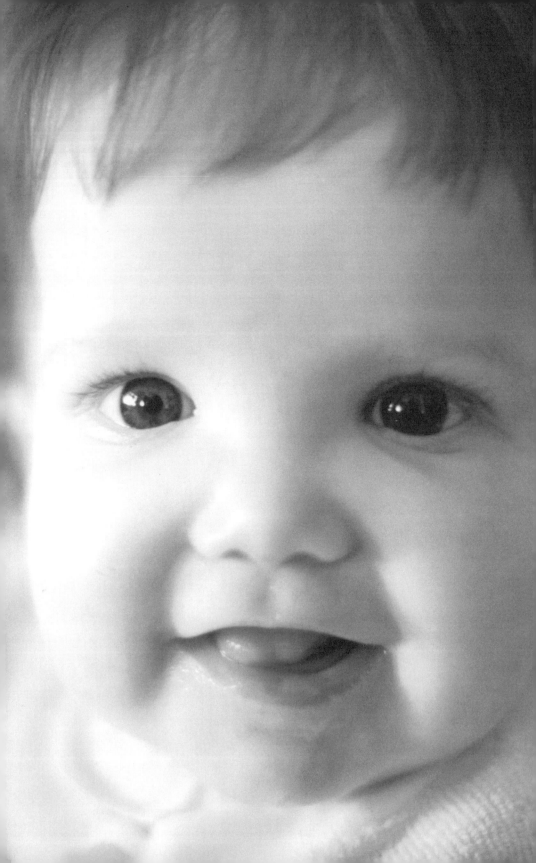

1

Awakening to the Soul of the Unborn

This book came as quite a surprise. One clear winter night sixteen years ago, standing gazing at the stars on top of Mount Madonna, California, sensing the stillness of the redwood trees around the cabin where my wife and I lived, the book sprang to mind in its entirety: title, outline, perspective, message.

Although I was extremely busy, working twelve to fifteen hours a day, I dropped everything and started typing. Seven intense days later, the manuscript was complete.

We were four months pregnant at the time. I had been doing "radiance exercises" with our unborn child, similar to those in this book, ever since we consciously realized that we had conceived.

Long before there was any physical bulge to demonstrate the baby's presence, we developed a marked spiritual bulge! I began to sense the child's spirit very strongly. This experience became more and more intense and coherent, and a close communion with the spirit of our unborn child developed. I became aware of the potential of this link. We could develop a relationship with the incoming spirit long before birth, and ease its transition into the world.

As the frequency and depth of my communication with the child grew over the next few weeks, I began to sense the character and intent of this spirit in a very specific way, just as you would develop a sense of the character and intent of a friend you spent a great deal of time with. I touched the identity of this being I was helping welcome into the Earth, and the purpose for which it had chosen to incarnate.

That night under the stars, I felt the spirit of this incoming one very close. In that state of still communion, it seemed I was tapping into the mind of the baby. In its mind I sensed, among other things, the desire to communicate to other parents the possibility of conscious prenatal contact with the fetus. The spirit of this baby wanted to explicitly lay out for other parents the practical steps they can take to get in touch with their children in the period of stillness that precedes birth.

Beyond that, *Communing With the Spirit of Your Unborn Child* has a broader message that applies to every person on Earth, not just parents-to-be. That message is that it is possible for us to be fully healed, to be fully who we are, that we can at any age assume the perspective of the eternal universal child, full of wonder, awe and innocence. We can move through the world, move through our lives with grace, unafraid, releasing a constant stream of blessing and healing to everything and everyone around us. It is never too late to be reborn! No matter what our physical age is, a small but radical change of perspective enables us to see, through a child's eyes, a fresh, magical world, full of the glory and beauty of newness. So in the last few chapters, there are some amazing exercises to help us heal our own childhoods, our own past, at any time in our lives.

What you will read is what I understood of the message I became aware of. I wrote the words as I sensed them in the moment. Whenever I was stuck for the next sentence, all I had to do is listen to the voices that spring from the silence within.

I am an unlikely person to write such a book. Though I have a strong and constant sense of spiritual guidance, I am not given to dreams, visions or visitations. Before the experience of connecting with the spirit of this child, I had a dread of parenting. I had little ability to relate to children; I could certainly not imagine enjoying them. The news that we were pregnant was not good news to me; it was like an unscheduled catastrophe, interrupting my pursuit of my life's work and further binding me into a relationship I felt was already dead. My only picture of parenthood was as an expensive, onerous and inescapable responsibility.

How wrong I was! Our baby son Lionel was a joy from the first. He came into the world not knowing even the basics of how to take care of himself. Yet he knew two important things from day one: how to love, and how to play. Other parents sometimes warned me about disasters ahead, like The Terrible Twos. With care and connectedness, they never happened to me. Lionel is now a teenager, and each stage of his development has brought new pleasure. Every week I talk with Lionel and touch Lionel, and feel a love and connection that never dims. Parenting has been the longest sustained joy of my life.

We also had a little girl, five years later, called Angela. As she grows up, she brings my attention again to the magic of each stage of childhood, reminding me of the spontaneity and innocence in myself. Coincidentally, the very morning I reviewed this text, they both cuddled with me in bed for a long time; we talked about the day ahead, and shared our sense of love of each other. Little Angela said, "Dad, you're the most wonderful daddy ever." Lionel hugged his agreement. Will this deep bonding last beyond fifteen, the age Lionel is now? I don't know, but it has so far survived the typical shocks and perils of an active twenty-first century life.

The ideas in this book do not seem revolutionary today. In the late nineteen-eighties researchers publicized the finding that a fetus's ears are developed at twelve weeks. We know that they dream in the womb, and we wonder what they dream about. The age at which we consider a fetus a sentient being keeps getting pushed back, as new research confirms that children can remember specific womb and birth experiences.

When this book first appeared, the social climate was quite different. Communicating with your unborn child was regarded as bizarre. People who had enjoyed such experiences didn't talk about them—and silence is the ultimate taboo.

When I began to lecture and appear on radio and television after the book's first publication, some interviewers were sympathetic and others were not. I remember one talk show host for a small AM station in the Southwestern United States. He told me—off the air only—that as a twenty-year-old fighter pilot in the Pacific theatre of World War II, while airborne on an operational mission, he experienced a presence that he knew was the soul of his child. He knew this even though the news that his wife was pregnant had not yet reached him from the mainland.

Another talk show host began his television interview with the words, "Now tell me, Dawson, what sort of a scam is this?" He went on to be unremittingly hostile throughout the interview, even when women in the studio audience described their own experiences of communing with their unborn children.

The first edition of this book helped legitimize these experiences for many parents. Since then, an increasing body of literature has emerged to validate the claims of the intelligence of the newborn. And people increasingly recognize that spiritual growth is the most important thing that can happen in their lives. Parenting is one of the most profound spiritual acts available to us. It combines the intense physical experience of pregnancy and birth with the intense spiritual experience of welcoming a soul into a body, and attuning our hearts with our own souls.

This act demands the highest degree of attention on the part of both mother and father. Yet our society provides few tools to help teach us how to be spiritual parents. This book is part of a whole new generation of support materials enabling the parent-to-be to take up the challenge of spiritual parenting, and assist in the development of a generation of people with the potential to renew our entire planet.

Rewriting the text years later for this second edition, I find that these ideas have stood the test of time in my life. I've written a new start to the book, talking about the importance of bonding, and about the reemergence of the Soul in our culture. And I've written a new ending, summarizing sixteen years of lessons from my son's life. But the book's essential exercises and practices remain unchanged. This book is today what it was when first published a decade and a half ago: a divinely inspired message of hope, full of gentle, practical tools for establishing a soul relationship with your children from the earliest possible moment.

My spiritual journey—and this book—would not have taken form without the guidance and inspiration of a group known as the Emissaries. Dedicated to "the spiritual regeneration of the human race," this quiet band of people has worked without fanfare for over sixty years to educate people in the basic tenets of spiritual literacy. Thousands of people have taken Emissary classes, which are focused on how to apply spiritual principles to every facet of your daily life. I have been immeasurably inspired by some of the people who find themselves drawn into this association. The principles they taught me are the basis for the methods in this book. You can obtain information about the Emissaries at www.emissaries.org. Emissary classes and centers, found around the world, can nourish and support your commitment to connecting with your own children.

If you ever lose the child that ought to dwell eternally in your heart, all you have to do is be silent, and deeply listen. You will find the fountain of youth springing forth from within the roots of your own being. Its dynamic flow has the power to renew and reinvigorate your reality, your past, your present and your future. You the child have a lifelong task of teaching and inspiring you the adult.

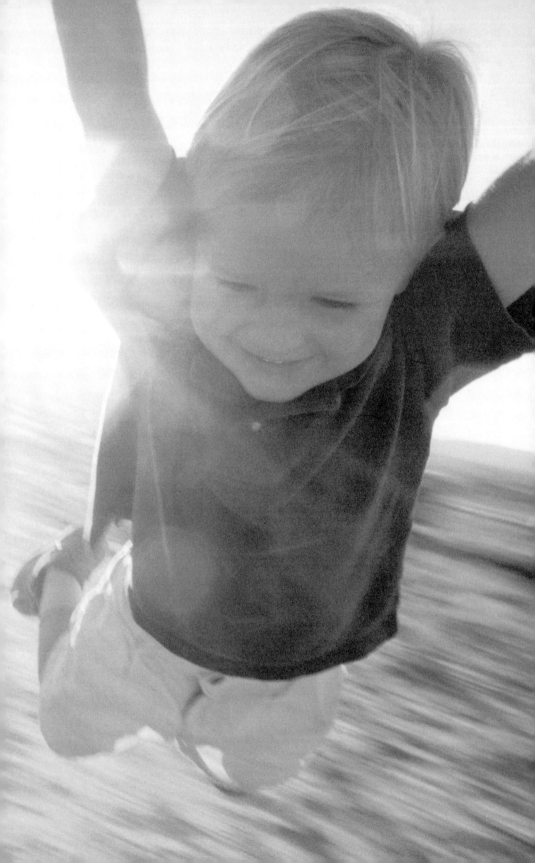

2

The Return of the Soul to Our Culture

Our culture's understanding of birth, and of the life of the unborn child in the womb, has undergone radical shifts in the last generation. Pregnancy and birth used to be regarded in western society as a medical event. Pregnancy was supervised by a medical doctor, as though it were a disease. Doctors became authority figures, deciding what births should look like, and in the case of caesarian sections, when they should occur. Doctors determined the experience of both mother and child to a large degree.

Birth moved. Instead of occurring in the bedroom or parlor of the home, it migrated to the hospital. It moved from the status of a family milestone to being a professional medical event.

Expectant mothers began to seriously question the prevailing norms in the fifties and sixties. Midwifery had never been quite stamped out, despite the best efforts of governments and doctors. Midwives began making a comeback; some began influencing or even running the obstetrics departments at hospitals. Home birth, water birth, husband-coached childbirth, and a variety of other organic alternatives began to catch on. Even the hospital environment changed. Many hospitals have banished stirrups, forceps and plastic sheets, and have now built special birthing rooms, complete with soft fabrics, low lighting, music, and bathtubs.

Alongside the changes in the physical environment for birth, parents, researchers and caregivers began to realize the effects of psychological and emotional health as well. Early studies showed that children exposed to classical music in the womb scored better on academic measures. Many other experimental studies have now been performed and replicated, showing a wide variety of effects that spring from early psychological conditioning. Parents with a rich verbal life produce children who develop vocabulary sooner. Parents who speak to their children in the womb produce better learners. Children in the womb may react distinctly to musical stimuli.

My son Lionel had distinct music preferences in the womb. When he was moving about rapidly, his movements would become slow and calm if Mozart or Bach were played. But he kicked violently on hearing Beethoven or Brahms, and didn't stop till the music had been turned off. Brenda and I had to leave a theater once, because the baby was kicking her painfully in the ribs as we watched a movie with a loud, discordant score by Prokofieff! Many parents have similar stories.

These discoveries led to a generation of products to facilitate learning in the womb; belts containing tape players, music CDs designed for the fetus, songbooks for the expectant mother, and many others. Parents realized that what they did with their children at this stage of development affected a child's subsequent life, sometimes in powerful ways.

Marriage of Psychology & Chemistry

At the same time, the science of endocrinology was coming of age. The effects of endocrine secretions were being mapped, and their sometimes-dramatic effects on both mother and fetus started to be understood. While blood and plasma do not travel between the mother's vessels and those of the placenta, many molecules can and do. One of the placenta's most important functions is to convey oxygen from the mother's blood supply to that of the fetus. But hundreds of other molecules cross the placental barrier as well.

Emotion is a biological event as well as a psychological one. When we feel good, our brains produce endorphins. Other glands and organs also produce hormones in response to pleasure, pain and every emotional state in between.

In one landmark study, a group of researchers studied the effects of spending five minutes in the morning concentrating on a powerful positive memory. They measured the body's output of Immunoglobulin-A, a factor associated with immune system function. People whose immune systems are functioning at peak levels have more Immunoglobulin-A in their bloodstreams than those whose immune systems are suppressed. The immune system itself is a useful benchmark, because it is composed of parts of the circulatory, nervous, skeletal and muscular systems, as well as the brain. By measuring immune system function, you have a summary of how well many other body systems are functioning.

They found that test subjects had a big immediate spike in the levels of Immunoglobulin-A in their bloodstreams after their five minutes of positive reflection. For the control group, who did not do the contemplation exercise, levels of Immunoglobulin-A stayed flat.

But the study did come up with one big surprise. The researchers found that, amongst the happy thinkers, levels of Immunoglobulin-A dropped only slowly in the subsequent hours, taking up to eight hours to drop back to the baseline level. Five minutes of positive contemplation produced a workday's worth of boosted immune system function! Tinkerbell was giving us a valuable piece of health advice to Peter Pan when she said, "Think your happy thought!"

Our thoughts and feelings, every minute of every day, together brew a powerful cocktail of mood-altering chemicals. Positive mental and emotional states produce marked effects in our bodies.

They similarly affect the body of the unborn child. When the mother is happy, the biochemistry of bliss is flowing through her veins, and from her into the baby's developing body. When the mother is upset or angry, the chemical messages are likewise passed along. The fetus develops in a biochemical stew determined largely by the mother's emotional and mental state. The fetal cells are literally bathing in this mix as they grow. And the combination of hormones brewed by the mother becomes of the imprint of what feels "normal" to each cell of the fetus.

This is why behavior doesn't start getting learned after birth. It starts long before the brain is distinctly developed in the fetus. The mother is giving even the first two cells of the dividing egg a biochemical message of what mix of hormones constitute the home signal. Tinkerbell might have told mothers to think happy thoughts for the sake of their babies' future happiness. No matter how close we get to friends, children, and lovers, none of us will ever have an emotional and psychological link to anyone in our entire lives that is closer than the one we had with our mother in her womb.

If a mother's heart and mind are filled with turmoil, these signals likewise transmit to the child. A fetus developing within a fearful or angry mother has the biochemical cocktail of stress running through its cells. Its cells divide in a broth conditioned by the chemistry of hate or anxiety. After birth, such psychological states feel normal to the infant, because they replicate what it knew during the formative period of its physical self. Upset mothers are creating a powerful program of upset conditioning in their children-to-be. Such conditioning is more than a psychological impression or "vibe"; it's biochemically hard-wired into the child's cells.

As the understanding of the effect of a mother's psychological state on the fetus has grown, women have begun to take care of their psychological health during pregnancy in new ways. Prenatal yoga classes have sprung up everywhere. There are endless relaxation tapes and baroque music CDs for pregnant mums. Pregnant women are to be found meditating in record numbers. They take more time off work before the birth. They encourage their children and their husbands to provide a quiet, calm emotional setting for the family. They go to therapists and support groups. They monitor their inner state for old habits of anger and fear, and when they are tempted to blame or condemn, they breathe instead. Doing this, they are giving their children the immense gift of an innate understanding of what inner peace "feels like" in a biochemical sense. For the child, knowing what the body feels like when the hormones of peace and serenity are flowing is a gift, a gift that benefits the child all life long.

The Third Great Leap

Parents reclaiming the birth experience from allopathic medicine formed a first great wave of change. Parents taking control of their own emotional space was the second great wave of change. We are now at the start of a third great wave, that goes beyond the physical birth environment, and beyond psychology: parents reclaiming the territory of the soul.

Over the course of the last thirty years, polls have revealed steadily increasing numbers of people identifying themselves as spiritual but not religious. As cultures have looked beyond their ancient religions for answers, Buddhism has taken firm hold in the western and northern parts of the globe, Christianity has grown in the east and south, and Islam has surged far beyond its historical crescent from North Africa to South East Asia. Many people claim no religion, yet report deep spiritual experiences.

Moving pregnancy and birth from a sterile ward to a more natural setting was an important first step. It reflects a greater attunement to the mother's body and the child's body. The next step is to consider the mother's heart and soul, and the child's heart and soul. How can we midwife the birth of a whole soul? Aware of our own spiritual journey, how do we relate to the spiritual journey of a child being born to us? We all ask ourselves the great existential questions, questions like, "What is the purpose of my life?"; "What is God's will for me?"; "What work is my soul looking to accomplish through me?"; "How can I give my spirituality meaningful expression in the world?"; "How can I know God" and so on. It's only a matter of time before we begin to ask these questions not only for ourselves, but for the children being born to us as well.

When I wrote the first edition of this book in the late nineteen-eighties, midwifery was catching on again, and there was an explosion of interest in alternative birthing techniques. But the deeper questions about the spiritual meaning of birth had not yet been asked. Today, many parents realize that taking care of their own souls is important. They are beginning to ask how to relate to their children on a soul level as well. Birth is as much a spiritual event as a physical event—perhaps more so. It may be one of the two or three most significant spiritual events in people's lives.

It is comparatively easy to educate yourself about the physical processes of birth. There are literally thousands of books, videos and web sites on the subject. You can understand the pregnancy process step-by-step, week-by-week, trimester-by-trimester. The territory is well know, the maps are many and accurate. The psychological territory is also being mapped in research like the Immunoglobulin-A study outlined above.

When you venture into the soul's territory, though, the terrain is vague and unknown, the data scarce, the maps partial and sometimes contradictory. How do you connect with the soul of a fetus? How do you know that any intuitive impressions you receive aren't just your imagination? Are there reliable methods of connecting with a baby's soul routinely, methods as clear as Tinkerbell's? Is communication with a soul susceptible to methods and techniques at all; is it not properly the misty province of seers and mystics? Where does soul-to-soul contact with my baby fit into my religion? Is the baby's soul well-developed enough to be able to communicate back to me?

My prediction is that, in the decades to come, we will map the territory of the soul as surely as we've mapped the physical features of the Earth or the psychological functions of the brain. Our understanding will always be incomplete, but for the next generation of parents it could seem inconceivable that we not ask the above questions, and foster soul-connection between parents and children.

This book's modest goal is to give parents easy yet effective techniques to allow contact with the soul of the child. You don't need great intuition or psychic powers. The instructions are paint-by-numbers simple. Yet I can almost guarantee that any parent who tries these methods will be surprised—if not awed—by the insights they obtain from their child in the womb.

The Soul in the Great Religi...

I've tried not to tie this book to any religion in particular. I was raised a Baptist, and thoroughly enjoy the church services at the Charismatic Episcopal Church, where my father and brother-in-law are both priests. I've learned a great deal about non-attachment from Buddhism, and I practice sitting meditation several times a week. The great cosmic archetypes of deity in Hinduism, and some of its forms of worship, speak to me. I've read a great deal of Jungian psychology, as well as other psychological schools. I'm indebted to The Emissaries for their marvelous classes, which while drawn primarily from the Judeo-Christian tradition, emphasize the Great Tradition that spans ever religion; what Aldous Huxley called the Perennial Philosophy.

I love Sufi dancing, poetry, and stories. Living in the United States for twenty-five years, I've inevitably read Native American wisdom and taken sweat lodges from traditional Indian medicine men. I've been a member of several churches, most recently Unity and Religious Science. I haven't found one of these spiritual practices that would fail to understand the concept of a soul, and there isn't much in this book that would conflict with any but a narrow fundamentalist interpretation of any of the above spiritual traditions. The same great truths run through the teachings of all the world's religions, and I try to reflect them in the following chapters.

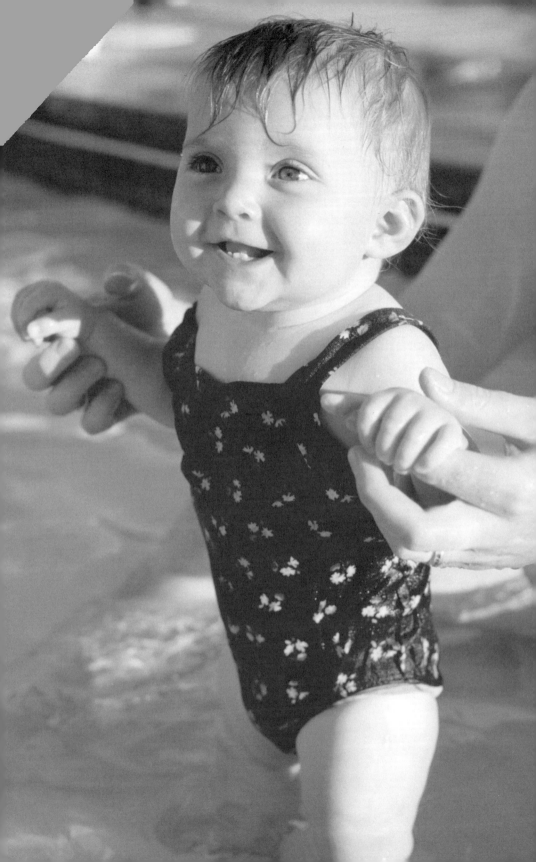

3

The Miracle of Bonding

Michelangelo's Pieta, Mary holding the body of Jesus, is an image that can never be forgotten once you have seen it. I've only seen pictures, never the real thing, yet the vivid white marble lines live etched in my brain forever. Likewise the image of the Madonna holding the child; from the mosaics of the Byzantine Empire, to the sweepingly modern minimalist ceramic figure I gave to my father one Christmas, the image of the mother and child has endless fascination. It's an image so primal, so archetypal, that you could show the image of a Black Madonna from the steppes of Catherine the Great's Russia to a Yanomami tribesman living in the remote depths of the Amazon rain forest, and the tribesman would immediately grasp the meaning of the image.

The image of the mother holding the child is so absorbing that I stare whenever I see it, whether it's a real live soccer mom navigating the aisles at Macy's with an infant, or a Zimbabwean sculptor's soapstone Madonna reposing in an upscale wine country gallery. The image compels attention.

Parents and children are bonded in the most powerful of ways. The act of carrying a child bonds that little human being to the mother forever—however loving or unloving the mother may be.

The bonding process is vital to the survival of our species. While a foal can walk beside its mother an hour after birth, while a baby humpback whale is swimming with the pod the same day it's born, newborn human beings are helpless for over a year. They require feeding, cleaning, transportation. They are born at a much earlier stage of neuromotor development than their mammalian cousins. Mother, father, siblings, grandparents, and other members of the tribe are essential to keeping them alive.

Without feeling bonded, mothers would never put forth such superhuman effort. Bonding is foundational to the human species. Men and women may bond in love relationships, people may bond in friendships or sexual relationships, but no other bond is as basic as the one formed by carrying a child in one's womb. Bonding is not something we have to do or create; it is inherent in the act of parenting. Parents don't have to take classes in order to learn how to bond; the word "bonding" describes something that is naturally present, that does not have to be created or learned.

Communing with the soul of your unborn child powerfully promotes bonding. Seeing the physical body of the baby pushing the mother's tummy may symbolize physical bonding. But becoming aware of the soul of the baby traveling to inhabit its new vessel engages levels of heart and spirit that bond parents to baby in a much deeper way.

Conventional psychology teaches that while mothers bond with children in utero, fathers don't begin to bond strongly until after birth. Men are more visually and physically oriented than women, and the sight of their newborn is considered by psychologists to be a prime bonding trigger. The baby becomes real to the man when he can see it, hear it, and touch it.

An immense gift of bonding with the soul is that it can be done equally by fathers and mothers. I had powerful experiences of becoming bonded with my children before birth, and I assume throughout this book that fathers will be as actively engaged in the process as mums. A father bonded with the soul of his child will be much more involved with the entire course of the pregnancy than a father who waits till after birth. A soul-sensitive father doesn't have to wait until the third month, or the seventh month, to bond. Bonding early, many months before the birth, gives the father a strong bond with the child by the due date. It's a gift to the mother to have a father present at the birth who is already powerfully connected into the triad of the new family. If the father is coaching the mother in breathing or posture, he will be much more sensitive to her and to the baby if he is strongly bonded. This contributes to an easier labor and delivery for both mother and baby.

Bonding with the soul can also be done by an entire community. Spiritual teachers can pray with the mother and father. Grandparents can lay their hands on the mom's belly and let their love pour in. Little brothers and sisters can picture a love-angel coming to live in mommy's tummy. The mother may feel the presence of invisible angels guiding, protecting and nurturing her. In this way, the mom never has the experience of facing a pregnancy and new arrival alone. A community forms around her, people bonded to both her and the baby.

Soul work opens up a completely new experience of parenting. Instead of pregnancy being the mother's lonely work, suddenly there are many invisible threads of support available to her. Soul-based parents have a basis and vision for parenting that embraces a far greater spectrum of human experience than those parents who consider only at the little body that is growing in the womb.

As you go through the exercises in this book, you will sense not just a fetus but a person. You will have a growing sense of what your child is like. After some practice, you will recognize the soul-signature of your baby as effortlessly as you would be able to pick out your spouse by scent and touch alone. You will find respect and admiration growing for this being. In fact, you might have the purest being-level connection with your child than you have in your entire life. This is because, later on, when you're dealing with diapers, sleep deprivation, and crying, it's often harder to tune in to the soul. The time in utero is a marvelous, sacred opportunity to connect at a time when both you and the baby can be sensitive to the soul work that is occurring, without the homework, bobby socks, video games, and other distractions that can quickly fill up the space of relationship as your children grow up. Make the most of it! And cast your net of loving, supportive community as wide as you dare!

PART TWO

Getting In Touch

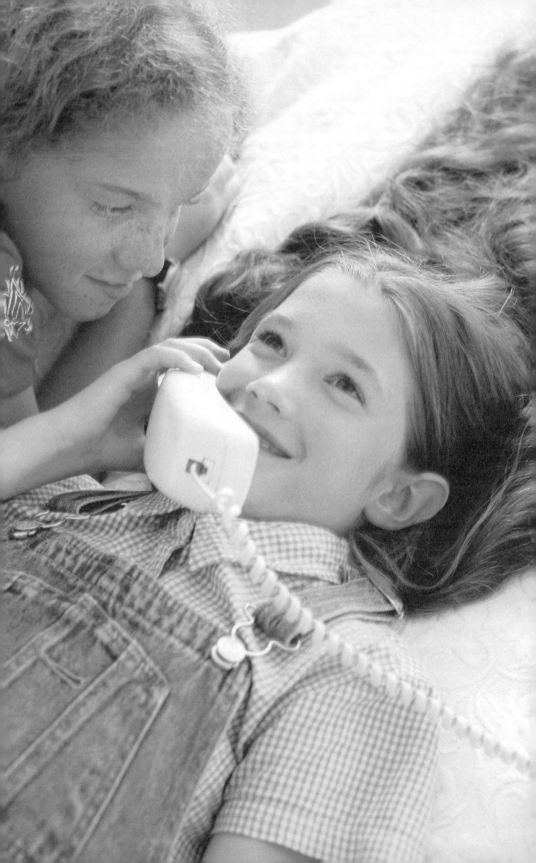

4

The Universe Is Speaking To Us

An old story tells of a great warrior who walked up to and old monk and demanded, "Teach me about heaven and hell." The monk responded scornfully, "How can you call yourself a samurai? Your armor is dirty, your sword is rusty, and you stink!" The warrior, outraged, drew his sword to strike off the old man's head. As he raised his arms over the frail figure, the monk stared deep into the warrior's eyes and said: "That's hell."

The warrior was pierced to the heart. He dropped his sword and fell at the monk's feet. "Forgive me," he sobbed, "for my arrogance and anger."

Fondly rubbing the warrior's head, the old man said, "That's heaven."

In every generation there have been teachers who, like the old monk, called the societies around them back to God. Every culture and civilization had its holy people, it's Gautamas, Moseses, Lao-Tzes, Jesuses, those very exceptional individuals who had not forgotten the heaven from which they came, and who devoted their lives to reminding the people around them who had forgotten their source.

While in times past there were a few masters, and a seeker might have to travel for many years and many miles to find a true teacher, today there are many. A great number of the children being born at this time in history are masters, come to usher in a new world.

Our planet functions as a living organism. It has a circulatory system in the oceans, clouds, rain and rivers; a respiratory system in the great tropical forests, and all the other characteristics of a living creature. In this planetary whole, humankind plays the role of the global brain, a communicator and integrator of information. Humans are the conscious component of Earth.

Up to this point in history, acting as though our species alone mattered, humankind has been destructive. Our species has been like a diseased organ, planetary rogue cells preying on the whole organism in order to gain those things we short-sightedly consider to be in our own interest. Life works in synchronized harmony throughout the cosmos. Only in this one, curious, deviant world do we find the dominant species creating conditions which are inimical to its own survival and the survival of the whole.

The universe has given us gentle reminders of wholeness and integration from time to time, in the persons of great teachers like the monk, teachers who have come to call our memory back from hell to heaven. Sometimes the societies into which they've been born have killed them. Sometimes they've deified them, rendering their message impotent by wrapping it in the shrouds of religious dogma.

In the past, such exceptional beings donned human guise only occasionally. No age could tolerate too many of them. But today, a whole new order of beings is incarnating on Earth, choosing to assume physical forms in order to assist the spiritual regeneration of our planet. The universe is gifting the Earth with souls appropriate for this stage of our development as a species. They are not subject to the limitations of the last generations. They are pushing at the boundaries of all cultural forms.

Today, with so many new children bringing the message, our ability to deafen our hearts has weakened, and we are collectively ripe for a shift in our underlying assumptions about the nature of the cosmos and our position within it. The unsustainability of the old way of doing things is becoming apparent to even the most intransigent minds.

A second Renaissance is occurring, a spiritual Renaissance that marks the defining watershed of planetary history. Books, movies, print and electronic media are reflecting this spiritual revolution. It has even reached the organized religions, sometimes the first to reject and the last to accept spiritual regeneration. Fundamentalists, traditionalists, orthodoxes, modernists and reformists are finding their hearts rekindled by the deepest teachings of their faiths. It is reaching into the heart of every religion on the globe, subversively using the very teachings at their cores, long buried under the grave clothes of liturgical ritual, to revitalize them.

If we teach our children using even the most advanced lessons of yesterday, we will miss the mark. The lessons they need to learn are radically different. The most enlightened of the nineteenth-century educational approaches are inappropriate for a twenty-first-century child. To use them is like hitching an ox wagon to a bullet train. The new wave of ideas these children bring is vital to our planet's survival, and must not be obstructed by the old forms of education.

So how do we as parents then take responsibility for stewarding these beings, guiding them? The most important education we can give them is instruction in the Perennial Philosophy, the enduring truths that the great masters have exemplified for us through the ages. If we as parents are able to represent the ways of life to them, and ground their minds and hearts in resonant connection with universal truths, the rest of education will follow.

The old way is characterized by unconsciousness: unconsciousness of the way that the patterns and rhythms of life operate in the universe. The new way is characterized by a conscious desire to be at one with the rhythms of cosmic and personal nature, to fit in with the larger scheme of things. Paradoxically, it is by fitting in to the whole that we discover the fullness of our individuality.

If we bring the innate order of the cosmos into practical manifestation by living lives which are true to its principles, we both fulfill our maximum potential as individuals and bring our personal worlds into the sphere of influence of the life-order. It is our day-to-day living that has the potential to link the part with the whole, the mundane with the sublime, the ordinary with the transcendent.

From Chaos to Cosmos

Look into the eyes of a newborn baby. There is a wisdom there, a connection with universal source, that is utterly present. Light streams from these beings.

As parents or guardians, our responsibility is to create a spiritual and physical climate that allows for the maximum shining of that light. In the bad old days, society tried in every conceivable way to smother that light after birth. Children were pushed through shortsighted processes of education and socialization. They were indoctrinated into something called a religion, the chief effect of which was to replace their inherent intimacy with God with the prevailing theological rituals.

The new parent rejects the approaches of yesterday in order to become a sacred nurturer of the light of the newborn. All parenting is sacred parenting. There is no part of parenting that is not inherently a sacred act. The parent has the responsibility of finding the means to allow free expression of the inner being of the child. Although the inherent potential dwells within the child, it is not conscious, and the task of the sacred parent is to provide an environment in which the child's light is respected. The conscious parent kindles the unconscious light in the child. Every parent has an unceasing responsibility to the child to be the light, to represent the light.

Any parent can make spiritual contact with a child even before birth, establishing a channel of connection, bonding and understanding. In the process the parent's own spiritual understanding deepens and matures.

Reinventing Earth

As these new teachers incarnate among us, they bring to the mass subconscious of humanity a measure of understanding and education in the processes of life. At present we are seeing an explosion of these global beings incarnating as newborns. The universe is speaking to us in the language of the future, and the words of the new language are our babies.

These newborns are a gift to us from the stars. They are the people of tomorrow. They will not be living their lives by the rules by which we live, our parents lived, or our grandparents lived. The divine impulse is reinventing the Earth, and with it humankind is being remade in its image.

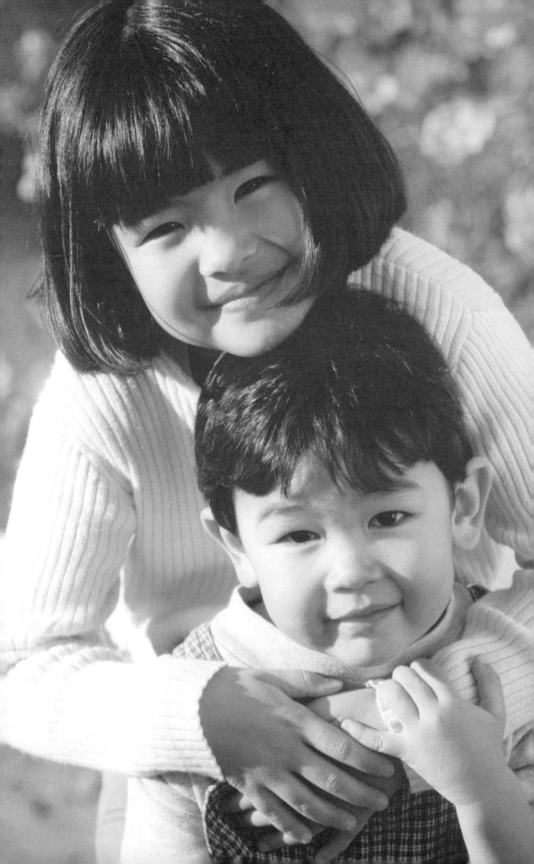

5

The Welcome

Sara was a forty-seven-year-old woman with waist-length salt-and-pepper braids. She'd been trying unsuccessfully to get pregnant for years. As she told me her story, sitting on a gray stone step in front of a fireplace at a conference center, playing with a happy young toddler on her lap, her eyes gleamed in the firelight. "I know the very night that we conceived," she said. "It was January 14th. My husband Alex had just come back from a weekend trip, and we had a fun, relaxed dinner together. Everything that night seemed happy and easy. When we made love that night, it was wonderful. The room seemed to me to be filled with a glow. I don't know how, but I just knew I had conceived."

Martha, an attorney, had a different story, "I didn't want a kid. My OB/GYN told me I was probably sterile, I hadn't got pregnant even though I'd rarely used birth control for many years. I'd just separated from my third husband when I missed my period, but I'm always irregular, so I thought, 'No big deal' and let it go. And my ex had a very low sperm count, so I was incredulous a couple of months later when a pregnancy test came back positive. I made the clinic test me three times, because I couldn't believe it. I felt this sick feeling in the pit of my stomach, because I knew I couldn't face an abortion and I was going to have a baby whether I wanted one or not."

The moment when a couple knows they are pregnant is usually a profound one. Suddenly there's a new world full of potentials and possibilities. Conception may be a long-hoped-for event, as in Sara's case. Or it may seem like an unforeseen calamity, as it was for Martha. Whichever it is, spiritual parenting demands of us that we have a very particular attitude at the instant we consciously know we have conceived.

This attitude is one of welcome. If our first flush of feeling is one of panic, of upset, of rejection, of dismay, this can imprint a subconscious pattern of rejection that endures throughout the development of our relationship with that child. If the feeling is one of rejoicing, of acceptance, of welcome, this creates a wonderful beam of energy on which the soul may travel in.

The child knows whether it is wanted or not. Just because the outer form of the child's mind is not yet developed does not mean that a certain level of knowing is not there. In spirit we know all things. We know things that are far beyond the comprehension of our conscious mind. When our identity is in spirit, things are known to us that go far beyond the scope of the perception of our conscious mind.

So our responsibility as parents begins the moment of conscious knowledge of conception. We may feel panic, dismay or uncertainty, but this our opportunity to transcend these feelings. Whatever cartwheels our emotions might do at the instant of conscious knowing, we have the ability to keep our spirit steady, radiating welcome and acceptance for this new soul.

This is the first great blessing we can offer our baby. It is the first spiritual gift we can give, establishing a precedent for the giving of other gifts.

We give thanks that a great spirit has consented to bless the physical form of our child with its presence, that it has chosen to incarnate through us. We give thanks that our love has provided the vehicle for the induction of a spirit that has come to bless the Earth.

Easing the Transition

A soul's transition to the physical plane is made easier if they know that the parents of the child through whom they are choosing to incarnate plan to do all that they can to make that soul's full manifestation possible.

When you go to visit a friend or relative, how do you view the upcoming visit? If you know that you will be given a royal welcome, that everything possible will be done by the ones who are receiving you to make you feel at home, accepted, at peace, you will look forward to it. If you know that they will be grumpy, preoccupied with their own selfish concerns, unable to be conscious of the larger world around them, you will probably view the coming visit as an ordeal.

The same thing is true at the soul level. If we can make the spirit of our baby feel welcomed, it will affect the entire incarnation. This is why at the instant of conscious knowing of conception, it is vital to roll out the red carpet in consciousness!

Shedding Heredity & Environment

I heard Ned's story at a party. "I had this rocky relationship with Nora, and I knew it could never be more than a short-term thing. She was unbelievably flaky, and I later discovered she'd tried every drug on the planet. She'd pop any pill anyone gave her in her mouth, just to see what effect it had. When she rang me and said she was pregnant, my first thought, was, 'Oh shit, I'm going be to stuck with this loser for eighteen years.' My second thought was, 'I know she sleeps around, I can't be the father.' So I demanded a DNA test, which showed that I was. I tried to get her to have an abortion, and we made several appointments but she either changed her mind or didn't show up. And I think she tried to have an abortion that I didn't know about, which was unsuccessful. I knew she'd be a disaster as a mother, and that if the baby was born it was going to be up to me to parent. This wasn't exactly the script I'd written for my life. My acting career was taking off, and I knew that a kid would make it impossible."

What about a situation in which the earthly parents are not happy to learn that they are pregnant? What about a case in which the parents don't want the child, and view it as an imposition, a nuisance, or a disruption?

Cassie was having an affair with a married man, Jim. She missed her period, which was always very regular. Two weeks later she had a pregnancy test and it came back positive. Jim came clean and told his wife about the situation that very day. However, Cassie had an extremely high level of anxiety about the situation. She didn't work for the three days, walking frantically around Central Park near where she lived on 60th street in New York during the day, and pacing her apartment during sleepless nights. She was frantic.

On the fourth day, she began to bleed heavily. She'd aborted spontaneously, probably linked to her very high level of anxiety about the situation.

Sometimes a soul that is placed in such a position by the prospective parents will not complete the incarnational process. This may take the form of a spontaneous or induced abortion, or a stillbirth. But usually the soul decides to come in anyway. The incoming child can overcome many things. Many of us may have had parents who were ambivalent, hostile or indifferent to our birth. If the soul believes it can accomplish its mission despite a lack of allies, it may enter the body of the baby anyway.

If you feel ambivalent about a pregnancy, don't make it about the baby or the other parent. Take a look at your own feelings. What fears do you have? What is the worst you think could happen? What is the best that could happen? Work these things through in your own heart, or with a counselor. A wonderful resource for sorting out these issues is *The Work* by Byron Katie. You can do the basic process on her web site, www.the-work.org, or use her book, Loving What Is. Her favorite quote is: "When you argue with reality, you lose—but only always."

A new baby is a big shift in your life, even if you have been wanting a child for years. It may well take time for your psyche to process and accept the reality of it. So if you're not immediately grateful, hold the idea in a neutral space for two or three weeks, to give yourself time to get used to your new reality.

Spirit can overcome all things. It can take the most nasty, twisted, problematic situations and turn them into triumphs. If we trust our inner sensing of our divine potential, even if we get absolutely zero reinforcement for this belief from the outside world or anyone in it, our connection with spirit can make our inner beauty manifest. Our dreams of our potential can come true. We do not have to remain limited by anything. We can always transcend our background. The inherent nature of spirit transcends the ways of the Earth. As soon as we become one with spirit, we transcend our past, and future too.

Margie is one of the most even-tempered people I know. I met her when we were both volunteering for an organization that helps homeless moms with kids. Margie is relaxed and cheerful; when you look into her eyes you see someone who is truly present. She works as a housekeeper and part-time midwife, drives a twenty-year-old Buick held together by rust and wire, and never has much money. Her mother was an alcoholic and her father abused and beat her. Her mother tried to have an abortion when she discovered she was pregnant with Margie Yet Margie has lived a life of inspiring other people with her lively eyes and good humor. When she describes her childhood, there's no emotional charge attached to the description; Margie's just stating facts without much emotional spin to them, and no expectation of sympathy or claim of victimhood. She believes that her upbringing helped her make different choices in her own life. Her goodwill extends to her only child, a pre-teen with whom Margie is very close. Margie helps her own child, other children, and her community. The bumper sticker on the back of her car says it all: "It's never too late for a happy childhood."

The reality of transcendence is available to you always. If you as parents did not give thanks at first, but have come later in the pregnancy process to an understanding of the imperatives of spiritual parenting, give thanks now, now that you have come into this knowledge. This process of giving thanks for conception is possible at any time. And the flood of blessing that is released when parents become thankful for their children can flood retroactively backwards in time to heal wounds present from the time of conception.

Even if that blessing was not there in linear time, it can be implanted in spiritual time. Spiritual time does not respect the boundaries of linear time. There are no limits to spirit. When it is given free reign, when it is allowed to flood into a situation, it overflows backwards in time to bless us from the point of conception. In the enlightened moment, every other moment is enlightened. In the moment of enlightenment, every other instant of our lives, past, present and future, is bathed in radiance. It overflows to everyone we know, everyone we have ever known, every one we will know in the future.

You may have parents that never gave thanks for your incarnation. But as you allow thankfulness to flood your being, you bless your own past. In this way you allow spirit to be your true parent, touching your own birth with the hand of healing.

Welcoming the Unknown

The following exercise may be done either to welcome in the spirit of your unborn child, or to welcome your own spirit now, which will welcome your spirit all the way to the time of your physical conception—however many years ago that may have been. Make yourself comfortable, in a quiet, darkened room. Make sure you will not be disturbed for about 45 minutes. You can read this exercise to yourself, or better yet, record it and play it back to yourself. You can also obtain a downloadable audio version of the book from www.Communing.com.

You may play some background music at low volume, something that is not distracting. If you have learned a specific meditative technique, meditate for a while before you begin the exercise. You know your own patterns and habits. Do whatever is necessary to make yourself completely relaxed.

§ § §

FIRST EXERCISE
THE DIVINE CHILD

Close your eyes. Breathe deeply. With each outbreath, visualize all the things that you worry about, that occupy your mind, that distract you from the present moment, flowing out of your body with the breath. Let your breathing become regular, and with each breath, expel a little more of the tension till your body is completely relaxed and your mind is still.

Breathe out, exhaling all the old, stale air from your lungs. Relax, and allow pure, clean, fresh air to be drawn back in. Breathe out and in several times in this manner. With each outbreath, feel the tension leave your body. As you breathe in, feel the fresh air streaming over your brain and mind, washing out all the preoccupations in your head. Let all your concerns, your worries, fade into the background. Let the cool, white, incoming air soothe your frustrations, smoothing over the rough patches in your life.

Visualize your body as being filled with green energy. This green energy is all the stored tensions that have been retained in your muscles and organs. See how this energy fills all of your limbs. Start at your feet. With each outbreath, feel the energy flowing out of your feet with the breath. Take as many outbreaths as required to clear out this green fluid from every nook and cranny of your feet.

Then go up your calves, thighs, pelvis, and work your way up. Take as much time as required to make sure that each part is completely relaxed. Turn off the tape until you have had time to release the tensions in every part of your torso. When you have completely cleared your shoulders of this fluid green energy, and each part of your body feels completely limp, see the energy that fills your head. Start at the back of your skull, and begin to expel it with each breath. Keep going till even the smallest cavities in your head have been emptied of the green energy, and no tension or tightness remains.

45

Finally, empty your neck and mouth of the fluid, and feel how completely relaxed your body has become.

Now let your attention review each part of your body again, to see if there are still any remaining pockets of the tension-energy. Find the subtle places where tension is still lingering, and allow it to flow easily out of you on the current of your breath.

Now as you breathe in, imagine a bright, glowing white substance, like mist. It is full of energy and life. Breathe it in, and feel it move to every part of your body, rejuvenating and soothing your muscles, your emotions, your mind. Let it smooth over all the bumps of worry and anxiety in your experience. Forget about all the problems you usually deal with, and feel your whole being invigorated by the experience of peace and vitality that it brings.

Think back to your first meeting with a child you really loved. It may be a brother or sister, or the child of a friend, or a child you only met once, but who filled you with joy. Whatever child it is, just remember how wonderful you felt being with that child: how beautiful that child was, how innocent, how fresh, how inspiring. Think of all the positive things you felt about that child. Remember all the feelings you felt when you were around that child. Give thanks for the presence of that child on Earth, wherever it may be right now.

Now picture the soul of that child. See the essences of spirit that came to focus in that child. Picture the great and profound presence that underlies that child's physical form. Blend with that presence. Give thanks for that presence.

Now picture that child's face blending into your own face, the face of yourself as an infant. See yourself as full of wonder as you remember that child-being. See all the potential in yourself that you saw in that magical child. Hold this strong image of yourself blending into all that was fine and perfect in the ideal child. Feel the great soul that is you coming in to that little body. Feel that magnificent soul fill that body with vibrant light, so that every cell sings with thankfulness. Feel the presence of God touching the child's body all around, protecting it from harm and hurt. Now imagine yourself as a younger child. Get younger and younger each moment until you see yourself at birth, and keep going. Feel what it was like to be in the womb. Feel how safe and snug it is, how secure you feel, how protected you feel from all harm. Enjoy float-ing in the fluid environment of this quiet place.

Keep on getting younger. Get smaller, as you go back in time to the first cells that were you, till you are only one cell. Then, from above, a bright light bursts in above you, a streak of lightning filled with love and purpose. It is spirit incarnating in your form. It fills you with purpose. Suddenly you feel you are heavenly, angel-ic. Experience yourself as part of both worlds: the cell, earthly, and the spirit, divine. Feel the exquisite tension of this dual nature.

Feel your soul giving thanks for the priceless opportunity to be incarnate. Your soul has been disincarnate for many years. Now at last it has the chance to be creative in form on Earth. And its first act of creation is to create you, the proto-fetus! You are the first creative act of love made manifest! You are filled with excite-ment and thankfulness.

Now, with this priceless knowledge firmly fixed in your aware-ness, this bliss of divinity, go forward in time again, as your cells grow and develop into a baby, then to birth. Bring this divine light to your own birth. Bless your birth with the wisdom and compas-sion of your own spirit.

Then move along to your childhood. Think of the wonderful times that you had, the achievements you were proud of. Let your divinity shine through those moments.

Now think of the worst incident you can remember as a child: the thing which terrified you the most; the most traumatic thing you experienced. Feel the way it felt. Re-experience all the agony.

Now bring your light, the light of spirit, to that situation. Comfort that grieving, ailing child. Bring the full force of your divinity to bear. Let the child feel your presence, feel that everything is all right. Smooth away the tears. Wash away the grief in the flow-ing river of your love. When the child is happy and comforted, move on to another such situation. Go through the process again. Comfort and sustain the child. As time goes on, you see your whole life in front of you, stage by stage. Wherever there was trauma, imagine yourself there, your divine self, with an endless supply of healing love. See how your soul guided your outer form to develop it to the point where you are today. Today you are able to see and actually experience the soul. This is the greatest miracle of all—that you can see and realize your oneness with your own divine self!

Your divinity is welcoming your body into manifestation. This divine presence embraces every stage of your life. It gives thanks for the miracle of your conception, birth and survival. You feel the immense sense of gratitude your soul felt at the instant of conception. You reach back and bless that instant now.

When you are ready to come back into your body, become aware of your breathing once again. Slowly become conscious of your inbreath and outbreath. Notice how relaxed your body feels, how refreshed you are. Become aware of the room you are in. As you get up and begin to move around, keep the feeling of thankfulness for being on Earth with you. Keep it present with you the whole day. Let it infuse all of your activities this day.

§ § §

This exercise is for use in preparing the consciousness of the adult who is initiating a connection with the child. Until our own attitude is right, our own heart is still, we do not have the ability to allow the fullness of welcome to flow through us to the baby. It is important to clear our own inner creative field of distractions, tension and limitations, otherwise part of our attention is siphoned off into these concerns, and we are not fully available to welcome our baby.

Once we have prepared our consciousness in this way, we are fully present and can bring our complete attention to bear on greeting the spirit of the incoming child. The next exercise is for use after you have completed the previous one. It focuses on the welcome itself.

The first three paragraphs of the following exercise are an abbreviated form of the relaxation technique which started off the previous one. If a period of several hours, or intense activity, elapses between using the two exercises, it is useful to use the longer form of relaxation found in the first exercise before proceeding to the second.

§ § §

SECOND EXERCISE
WELCOMING THE SOUL

Close your eyes. Breathe deeply. With each outbreath, visualize all the things that you worry about, that occupy your mind, that distract you from the present moment, flowing out of your body with the breath.

Let your breathing become regular, and with each breath, expel a little more of the tension till your body is completely relaxed and your mind is still.

Now as you breathe in, imagine a bright, glowing white substance, like mist. It is full of energy and life. Breathe it in, and feel it move to every part of your body rejuvenating and soothing your muscles, your emotions, your mind. It smooths over all the bumps of worry and anxiety in your experience. Forget about all the problems you usually deal with, and feel your whole being invigorated by the experience of peace and vigor that it brings.

Hold your hand over the pregnant uterus. Feel the presence of the child within. Feel the energy that emanates from the child to your hand. Feel your own spirit radiating back to the child. Feel the interplay of appreciation between the two of you.

Picture the details of the child's body, even though it may only be a fetus a few weeks old. Picture its head, its torso, its limbs. Now picture a glowing light in the middle of its chest where its heart is. See the love that is in that heart. Your own heart starts to glow with a sympathetic resonance. Your heartbeat synchronizes with the heartbeat of the fetus.

Now picture a ray of brilliant white light reaching up from your shared glowing hearts up into the heavens. It is the beacon that will guide the spirit into the body. This is your signal to the soul that it is welcome, that you are ready and waiting for it. This brilliant light illuminates the soul's path so that it may find the child's body.

As the soul comes down the light-pathway to the body, a cloud of love and power descends. You can feel its presence. The baby can feel its presence. You feel your own body respond to the soul of the child with love and welcome. Thank the soul for choosing to incarnate. Give thanks for the role you played in making this incarnation possible.

As the soul blends with the child's body, the beam of light gradually fades and becomes less focused, until it is just a glow which surrounds the baby. With this glow of protection hovering all around the child, you become aware of your breathing once again. You feel yourself breathing in and out, in and out, in and out. You have a tremendous sense of well-being. Your body feels refreshed and renewed.

Return your awareness to the room you are in. The sense of thankfulness will stay with you the whole day. At any time of this day you choose, you can feel your link to the baby as a glowing white cord that connects you. Along this cord, love and blessing flow. Every time you remember the baby throughout this day, allow your sense of thankfulness, welcome and appreciation to flow along this cord.

§   §   §

It is never too late for a welcome. At whatever moment you learn to give thanks for the wonder of your own birth, for the wonder of your child's birth, you have given spirit thanks for coming into the world. As spirit is welcomed into the world it fills the world, and the world is transformed.

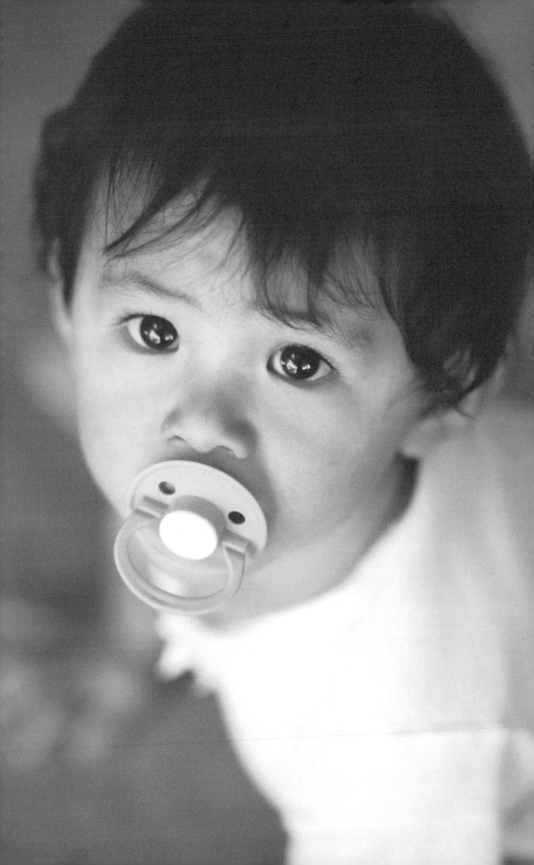

6

The Womb

The womb, in a physical sense, is a place where gestation of the material form of the child takes place. It is a place of protection. In it, the processes that create physical life are allowed to take form unhindered. In it, a new being may grow and come into manifestation in safety. The womb is an extraordinarily effective system for cushioning the developing fetus from the jars and shocks of the outside world. It is a safe place into which nothing can enter that does not belong in the burgeoning of physical life.

From conception to grave, the womb is probably the safest place any of us will ever be. Once we leave it, all kinds of perils threaten. We may find ourselves at the mercy of the capricious whims of an arbitrary society, whose rules are not the rules of the kingdom of life. In the womb, our innate beauty and creativity is not stifled, as it so frequently is during childhood. On the contrary, our innate perfection is free to express itself and become manifest.

Given this contrast, it is no wonder that, during regressive therapies such as hypnotherapy, patients weary from study at the school of hard knocks often dream of going back to the womb. It's not the literal, physical womb that is missed so much as that feeling of safety.

Japanese bonsai trees may be only a foot high when fully grown. They are kept small by tightly wrapping their branches with wire. Their growth is suppressed by constantly plucking out the growing tips of the branches. They are twisted into the forms deemed most pleasing by the gardener.

Inherent in each seed is the pattern of the full-grown plant. If seeds are allowed to mature without distortion, the full-grown plant reveals the beauty and glory that was potential in the seed. If, however, as the plant is growing, rocks are piled on top of it, or its developing branches are twisted and deformed by outside agents, the finished form does not reveal the full potential that existed in the seed.

This same process happens to most children. Their initiative is plucked out of them by an educational system that emphasizes rote learning, a device designed primarily to make it easy to classify large numbers of children by means of grades. Their growing forms are twisted by parental expectations, by peer pressure, by the arbitrary phobias of a mad society; by work, marriage, government policies, and all the other pressures of our time. No wonder we look back on the womb with nostalgia. It was a precious time of unfettered growth, before the deluge of distortions abruptly hit us.

Seeing Past the Veil

Think, for a moment, of another world. This world provides the same sense of safety, of nurturing your growth, that the womb provided. In this ideal world, that protection extends your whole life long. The whole of your life is lived in a womb of love. Instead of your innate beauty being distorted and blasted by the malevolent winds of the outside world, it is encouraged to grow into full bloom. Every person blossoms in his or her own way. No one is beaten down, denied expression, distorted by the expectations of others, or forced into the mold of a conformist culture.

This imaginary culture embodies the Spirit of the Womb. Each individual is allowed to flourish in his or her own way. The glorious potential of each one is unlocked. Society is enriched by the full release of each individual's special gifts.

As our understanding of the process of fetal development has grown over the last few years, we have come to realize that certain sensations get through to the womb. Prenatal psychologists have begun to turn up stories of people who, years later, remember things they could only have heard in the womb. The fetus does not abruptly begin to absorb sensory experiences once it leaves the womb. Its senses are functioning long before birth, busily receiving messages from the outside world.

As our spiritual understanding increases, we likewise come to realize that as well as being permeated by physical-level phenomena such as sound waves, the womb is permeated by spiritual and invisible forces. Emotions and thoughts can reach right through the physical flesh to touch and influence the growing fetus.

Vision of the Inner Eye

Because we as a culture are concerned chiefly with the physical and outward manifestations of things, we have tended to look at everything, including birth, from that level. As we move to the next level, as we metamorphose in consciousness into Homo spiritus, spiritual humans, we become aware of the spiritual dimension, and how it underlies and permeates the physical level.

We no longer see human beings merely in terms of their outer forms. We see the inner reality of things. We no longer rely on our physical eyes as our primary source of information. We see with the eyes of spirit, often noticing subtleties far beyond the scope of our physical senses. We may see something as being so, even though our physical eyes say it is not so. When the physical eyes look at the acorn, they see only an insignificant speck of matter. Seen with the eyes of spirit, though, potential is revealed, and the glorious oak tree is evident.

We similarly become aware that the physical level of the womb is not the end of the story. It is the beginning. It is underlaid with a greater reality: the Spirit of the Womb.

The Spirit of the Womb embraces all those qualities which we associate with the physical womb: safety, security, peace, stillness, growth, protection. The Spirit of the Womb is the place in which the processes of life are held inviolate.

The most memorable wedding I ever attended was one in which there was only one person at the altar. He was a thirty-two-year-old man called George. George had Down's Syndrome, and indeed by reaching the age of thirty-two, he'd already beat the odds of early death associated with this condition. He was small of stature, with a round, oversize forehead, bulging eyes, limited verbal skills, and all the other physical characteristics associated with Down's Syndrome. I'd been drawn to him at church services, and he to me.

In this wedding ceremony, George married himself. He'd conceived of, and planned, the whole event. The sixty guests were entertained by poi-tossing fire dancers, a cheerful Celtic music ensemble, and plenty of food. At the climactic moment, George walked up to the front of the hall, and sat on a throne-like chair. One of his caretakers read the vows he'd written: to be true to himself, to enjoy life fully, to love to the greatest of his ability. By the end of the ceremony there was hardly a dry eye in the room.

Despite handicaps you or I can barely dream of, George created a community of support for his own development. Without any money, living in a state-run group home, he'd managed to truly find himself, make friends, engage the people around him, and welcome himself into the world in a big public ceremony. He'd created his own womb, against formidable odds, and his wedding ceremony was a moving welcome of his spirit into the world.

Every pregnant couple has the responsibility for the creation and maintenance of a place of spiritual safety and acceptance for the soul of the baby. It is the responsibility of the male as much as it is for the female. Looking at a pregnant couple, physical level vision would judge the woman to be the one having the womb. When we look through the eyes of spirit and become conscious of the Spirit of the Womb, we realize that both the man and the woman are responsible for carrying and maintaining it.

Becoming the Peacekeeping Force

The man has a particular responsibility in this regard. While the woman has a primary responsibility on the physical level, the man has a primary responsibility on the spiritual level. The Spirit of the Womb is a place he carries within himself, with which he exercises great care. This involves not allowing negative or destructive thoughts and emotions to enter in.

Un-whole thoughts blow through the consciousness of each person, coming from our own subconscious, from the mass consciousness, from past or present circumstances. Yet we can choose not give them a home in our psyche. We have the option to say, "No!" We can allow such thoughts to move through us, not resisting or denying them, but certainly not harboring them.

For example, a man may have judgments about his partner, like, "I hate when she rests her foot on the clutch when she drives," or, "I wish she'd dress prettier," or, "She's tired again, I guess that means no sex for the second straight week," or, "If she only stopped talking," or, "Do we have to go to her Mom's house again," or any one of a million other irritations. During pregnancy, with consummate care for preserving the Spirit of the Womb, a man can take the care to notice such judgments, and not allow himself to react to them.

Those situations that grate on us the worst are the very ones in which it is most important that we maintain our inner stillness. Aggravations, in fact, are life's way of telling us: "Here is an area that needs attention, in which the power of peace, harmony and joy is absent. I am presenting this circumstance to you to enable you to change your unthinking, habitual behavior. I am showing you this so that you can cease exploding these spiritual bombs that so disturb the patterns of creative unfoldment in your own life and the lives of those around you. This irritation is my way of bringing this unhealed part of yourself to your attention, so that you may bless and heal it." If we seize the opportunity to change, our patterns are altered and our lives may be healed. The things that annoy us most are actually our most powerful paths to healing.

Preserving the Spirit of the Womb is something that is done in your own mind and heart. You are choosing not to express certain behaviors that are inconsistent with spiritual safety. You create the womb inside yourself, a place of serenity and safety in which your own spiritual potential and that of your child may grow. It is a carefully controlled environment in which to nurture creativity, joy, welcome, and peace.

When a parent takes responsibility for his or her own thoughts, creating an atmosphere of love around the family, he or she sets up a safe place in which life can bloom. The Spirit of the Womb is a sacred sanctuary in the hearts and minds of the parents.

The following exercise can help you get in touch with the Spirit of the Womb. Do it in a darkened, silent room, either alone or with your partner. Make yourself completely comfortable before you begin. If you've downloaded the audio version of this book, play this exercise softly. Otherwise, record the text and play it back, or have your partner read it softly and gently to you.

§ § §

THIRD EXERCISE
TOUCHING THE SPIRIT OF THE WOMB

Feel how comfortable your body has become. Feel the rhythm of your breath as you breathe in and out. Slow your breathing gradually. As your breathing becomes slower and deeper, imagine all the tensions of the day leaving with each breath. As you breathe and breathe, your body becomes soft and limp as all the tensions leave.

Breathe out, exhaling all the old, stale air from your lungs. Relax, and allow pure, clean, fresh air to be drawn back in. Breathe out and in, in this manner, several times. With each out-breath, feel the tension leave your body. As you breathe in, feel the fresh air streaming over your brain and mind, washing out all preoccupations. Let all your concerns, your worries, fade into the

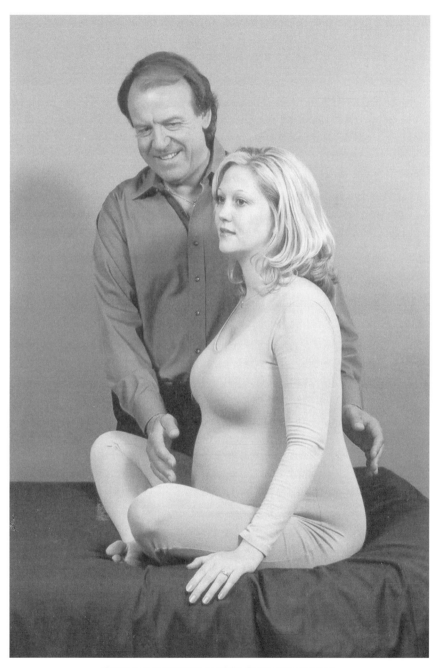

Getting an Initial Sense of the Spirit of the Womb

background. Let the cool, white incoming air soothe your frustrations, smoothing over the rough patches in your life.

Visualize your body as being filled with green energy. This green energy is all the stored tensions that have been retained in your muscles and organs. See how this energy fills all of your limbs.

Start at your feet. On each outbreath, feel the energy flowing out of your feet with the breath. Take as many outbreaths as required to clear out this green fluid from every nook and cranny of your feet.

Then go up your calves, thighs, pelvis, and work your way up. When you have completely cleared your shoulders of this fluid green energy, and each part of your body feels completely limp, see the energy that fills your head. Start at the back of your skull, and begin to expel it with each breath. Keep going till even the smallest cavities in your head have been emptied of the green energy, and no tension or tightness remain.

Finally, empty your neck and mouth of the fluid, and feel how completely relaxed your body has become.

Now let your attention review each part of your body again, to see if there are still any remaining pockets of the tension-energy. Find the subtle places where tension is still lingering, and allow it to flow easily out of you on the current of your breath.

Hold your hand or hands about twelve inches above the uterus. Visualize the child within. Imagine you can see clearly, using the eyes of spirit. Picture your baby's body. With your hand hovering above, you can sense what is going on in the womb. What sensations can you feel in your hand?

Now picture a bubble around your baby, extending a foot or more from the baby's body. This is the spiritual womb in which the soul is drawing together the vibrational substance which surrounds the baby as it grows. What color does it seem to be predominantly? What other colors are present? Is it moving? Pulsing? Or is it still?

Now visualize sending a current of radiant light from your hand to the bubble around the baby. Picture this stream of blessing pouring forth from you to the baby's spirit. Does the baby respond in any way? If not, fine. If it does, what does it do?

Move your hand over the surface of the bubble, touching it in each part, as you would caress a child. You are caressing the child's energy field. You are smoothing out the rough edges, and giving love and affirmation through your hand. You are welcoming this soul into the world. Let the full force of your love move through your hand. Feel the intensity of the moment increase as you pour your love out upon the child. Feel its love coming back to you, moving back to you through your hand. Feel the intensity increase as you exchange love with each other.

Sense the greatness of spirit that lies behind the baby. Give thanks to that soul for blessing this body with its presence. Give thanks for the moment of conception. Feel the love and lightness that you feel now travel back along the entire developmental path of the fetus to conception, enfolding it with love at every step it has taken to this point. Visualize this loving enfoldment of the Spirit of the Womb extending to the future, to a safe and loving birth. Picture the child, from month one to month nine, safe in the spiritual womb of love that you are providing.

Move your hands gently in and out, in and out, as though you are expanding and contracting the bubble. Feel the energy pouring forth from your fingers and into the bubble, as you love and bless the child. Keep your hands on the edge of the bubble, wherever you feel this is. If you feel that twelve inches is too close, move your hands further away until you find the correct distance that

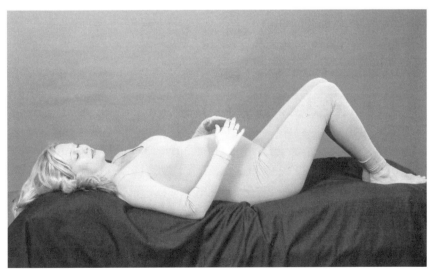

Sensing the Spirit of the Womb, Mother Only

defines the edges of your bubble. Keep that love and affirmation coming out of your fingers.

Now, gradually, move your hand further and further away, keeping the same feelings of love and appreciation flowing. Become aware of your breathing. Slowly become aware of your body, and how relaxed and refreshed you feel. Become aware of the room, and of the peace that fills it.

When you are ready, open your eyes and look around. Become aware of where you are. Look at your hand. Remember that whenever you see that hand, for the whole of today, you will remember the love and blessing that flowed through it. It will bring to your memory the Spirit of the Womb. You will remember the love you have for your baby, and the love your baby has for you. You will not forget this feeling, for you have something as close as your hand to remind you. Every time you look at your hand, you will feel love and thankfulness pouring forth from you into your child.

§ § §

Once you have touched the Spirit of the Womb and discovered the sanctity that accompanies it, you will probably not want to leave that space. You will want to maintain that spirit wherever you are, whatever you are doing, for the rest of your life. For the child you are really nurturing is the child within you. Your external child is simply an icon that represents the spirit of your own inner birth. We are given constant opportunities for new birth in every moment.

This exercise is one you can recall throughout the day to remind you of the Spirit of the Womb. Maintaining this calm spirit in the midst of our busy lives requires a level of spiritual discipline uncommon in our culture; however, pregnancy may give us great incentive to cultivate it. The incoming soul can make enormous progress if it is consciously aided by parents intent upon providing it the vibrational space in which to do its work. And our world is ready for the impact of facilitated souls. By becoming aware of the Spirit of the Womb, we give our whole planet a great gift.

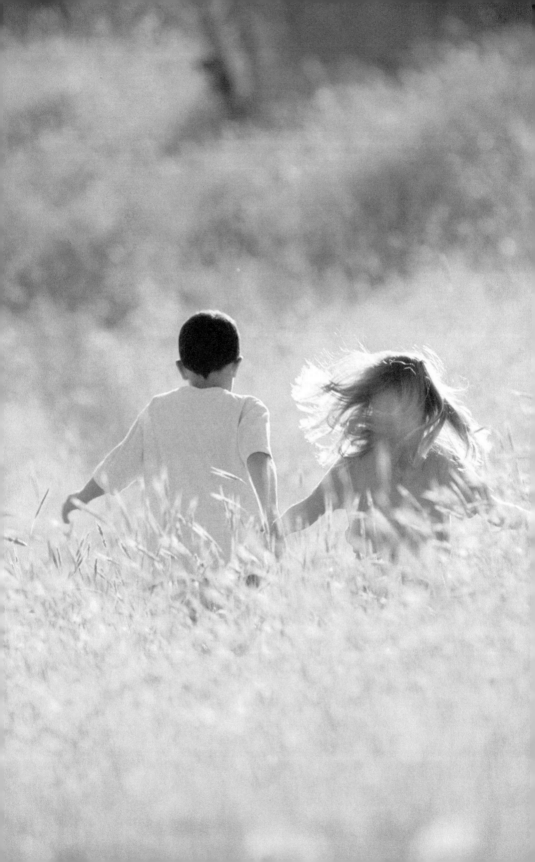

7

Sensing the Spirit
of the Fetus

J ust as individuals differ widely in their physical characteristics, emotional habits and mental patterning—the outer levels of being, there are similar differences in the spiritual character of each person—the inner levels of being. You are the person with whose outer levels you are most familiar. You are also very familiar with the outer levels of your partner, and if you have sought to understand the nature of your relationship on the inner levels, you have probably formed a sense of the spiritual identity of your partner as well.

By having a baby, you are inviting a third set of inner and outer characteristics into the equation. You become a triad, which creates a whole new configuration of spiritual energy.

Inner and Outer Dimensions

The outer levels are the body, mind and heart. In the world as we know it, outer bodies grow and become full-sized, so there is obvious development at the physical level. We also develop our minds, to at least some small fraction of their full potential.

Then we have the heart. We are usually educated to experience just small part of the vast emotional range of which we are capable. We think in terms of broad emotions such as love and hate, which is like knowing two chords on the keyboard of a piano. With such a brief repertoire of emotional experience, we are never going to make varied, interesting music. With hundreds of thousands of notes available, no two people need ever sound the same note twice if they are attuned to the delicate gradations of emotion that are possible.

When these outer capacities of body, mind and heart—the vehicle—are under the control of our spiritual or inner nature—the incarnate one, they can be used to express spirit, and manifest spirit. But when they are running the show, they are unavailable for the expression of spirit's purposes.

In the process of birth, spirit draws together a physical form, with its mental and emotional components, in order to incarnate on Earth. Each discarnate soul, in preparing to come to this plane, sets up for itself the combination of circumstances most suited to the lessons it has decided to learn and the purposes it has chosen to fulfill in the great creative scheme of things.

This transcendent aspect of each person, this divine spirit, manifests the outer form for its use. The outer form is the vehicle for the incarnation. It is rather like a car which the driver has put together to get him from point A to point B. The soul is the driver; the bodymind is the car. When this outer form of bodymind is responsive to the driver, the whole combination moves from point A to point B quickly and easily.

When, however, the chassis decides it wants to go one way, the engine decides it wants to go another, and the transmission a third, and none of them wants to fulfill the directives of the driver for whom they were built, chaos results. Put several billion discordant beings on the planet at the same time, and the whole world runs out of the control of spirit, going in disharmonious and destructive directions. Out-of-control cars tend to get pretty dented and bashed about, which is precisely what happens to the human divorced from being. It is the being aspect of human beings which makes us fully ourselves. The incarnational vehicle must be responsive to spirit in order to move with the creative flow.

Education for Seven-Dimensional Life

A child who is nurtured on the inner levels of spirit has an immense advantage over those who aren't. If we are not taught to honor spirit when we are children, we may teach ourselves later, but the process is apt to be full of collisions and traumas. If, on the other hand, children are raised under the sovereignty of spirit, the chances of their incarnational vehicles being under the control of the soul is much greater.

You will not become acquainted with the outer levels of the child until the child is born, and later. You will find out about your child's body, mind and emotional realm as these aspects develop. Underlying the outer levels are the inner levels, and these you can sense long before the physical form of the child is visible. Things of the outer are discerned using the outer capacities, while things of the spirit are spiritually discerned. Using your spiritual discernment, you can be aware of the spiritual characteristics of the soul that has chosen to incarnate in the body of your child long before birth.

A woman may sense the presence of the soul long before she meets a mate. "I see baby energy hanging around you," a psychic told Kath, a friend of mine. "I know," replied Kath, "But I'm being very careful because I haven't found the right man yet." A woman may feel kinship with a soul years before the physical mechanisms are in place for that soul to incarnate. This awareness can be thought of as spiritual conception; sometimes it happens many years before physical conception.

Some souls are reluctant to incarnate at all, knowing the challenges they will face on the Earth plane and the agonies their outer identity will go through before it discovers the being within. There is always the chance that these problems will so distract the bodymind that it never awakens to the presence of the soul within.

67

The Source of Education

Parents who are conscious of these hurdles can make a vast difference. They can smooth the path of the incarnating soul by giving the outer form conscious conditioning, predisposing the bodymind to awaken easily to the presence of the soul within. Parents unconscious of their responsibility can so load the bodymind with distractions and distortions that the awakening process is protracted and painful.

This is where spiritual-level sensing is so vital. Parents cannot learn what their child will require by reading child psychology textbooks. *Parenting* magazine is no substitute for spirit-filled parenting; Dr. Phil's advice is no substitute for spirit-filled relationships!

Your child may have requirements that defy textbook wisdom. Trust spirit; trust your inner knowing; get in touch with what your child is saying to you from the womb. It does not hurt to read and to consult authorities. This can be very useful. The creative process often picks up bits and pieces of knowledge from the outside world in order to tell us something.

But the knowledge stored in your mind or in books or in other people's minds, even those of experts, should not dictate what we do. Guidance should come from spirit. Educated people are no better at sensing spirit than those whose outer minds are less cultivated. Brilliance of mind is no advantage. Truly brilliant people are those who have yielded to spirit, whose behavior is controlled by the urges their deepest truth. Spirit controls their actions.

If we've educated ourselves in the school of spirit, we have worlds of knowledge at our fingertips. Just as our muscles grow as they are used, our sensitivity to spirit grows as we employ it, and we may find ourselves wise beyond our experience. We need strong spiritual bodies for the task of parenting angels.

Tuning In

As you begin to tune in to your baby, your perceptions may be faint and indistinct at first. The clutter of the mind may be loud, and hearing the channel of spirit may be like searching for a whisper on a radio dial full of raucous channels.

Don't despair! Inner sensing becomes stronger and more precise with use. We aren't taught these sensitivities as we grow up, so we tend to grow up without developing them. The advent of a new baby is a great opportunity to begin to develop our faculties of spiritual perception. And this sensitivity will allow our baby to communicate its needs to us.

My twenty-something friend Nan was expecting a baby. She was a vegetarian. Nan did more than practice; she was a passionate and committed advocate of vegetarianism. When she began to channel the spirit of her fetus, she felt the spirit of the child pushing her strongly to eat meat! Lots of it! And red meat! Her voice rang with outrage that I could hear even over the phone as she told me her story. Nan realized that to work with her baby she had to abandon her cherished ideals, at least for a while. As she began to eat meat during the pregnancy, her tendencies toward low body weight, fatigue and anemia disappeared. Both she and her son were in vibrant health when she finally gave birth to him.

The following exercise may be used to contact the spirit of the fetus. Before you begin, put yourself in a physical environment that is still and free of distractions. A darkened room may be helpful. Play, at very low volume, some soothing music. You can have a friend or your partner read you the exercise, you can record it and play it back, or you can download it from www.Communing.com. Have some paper handy so that you can write down your experiences once you are done.

§ § §

FOURTH EXERCISE
THE NEEDS OF THE FETUS

Close your eyes. Breathe out, exhaling all the old, stale air from your lungs. Relax, and allow pure, clean, fresh air to be drawn back in. Breathe out and in, in this manner, several times. With each outbreath, feel the tension leave your body. As you breathe in, feel fresh air streaming over your brain and mind, washing out all mental preoccupations. Let all your concerns, your worries, fade into the background. Let the cool, white incoming air soothe your frustrations, smoothing over the rough patches in your life.

Visualize your body as being filled with green energy. This green energy is all the stored tensions that have been retained in your muscles and organs. See how this energy fills all of your limbs. Start at your feet. On each outbreath, feel the energy flowing out of your feet with the breath. Take as many outbreaths as required to clear out this green fluid from every nook and cranny of your feet.

Then go up your calves, thighs, pelvis, and work your way up. When you have completely cleared your shoulders of this fluid green energy, and each part of your body feels completely limp, see the energy that fills your head. Start at the back of your skull, and begin to expel it with each breath. Keep going till even the smallest cavities in your head have been emptied of the green energy, and no tension or tightness remain.

Finally, empty your neck and mouth of the fluid, and feel ho completely relaxed your body has become.

Now let your attention review each part of your body again, to see if there are still any remaining pockets of the tension-energy. Find the subtle places where tension is still lingering, and allow it to flow easily out of you on the current of your breath.

You are now an empty form, limp and flaccid. Behind you, though, you can sense the presence of another being. This other being is a beautiful, shining presence. It is nothing but love for you. Its presence enfolds you, and you melt into it. In the bubble of its presence, you know that you are perfectly safe. In its presence you are at home. It welcomes you into itself, and your heart can rest in the knowledge that you have come home. You are free, safe and secure. You feel an upsurge of thankfulness that you have contacted this being, who is your true self, at last. Your years of wandering are over, and you can rest in the peace of having found yourself.

Feel how perfect this being is, how beautiful. Feel how there is nothing in the bubble of energy that is this being that could possibly threaten you, disturb you or upset you. It is fully you. It is truly you. Look and see the appearance of this being that is your true self. Notice the gorgeous colors, the perfect shapes. Spend as much time as you like just appreciating the wonder of this being. Notice details about its form, and how it flows. Merge every part of yourself with it in ecstatic union.

Now take time to look around you, around you two-who-have-merged-into-one. Notice that there is another such being of light. It is the true being of the one who is closest to you, of your partner in love. Notice how perfect the essence of your partner is. See your partner coming slowly towards you, till your light-forms are close to each other.

Notice those things that were special to you the first time you saw your partner. Notice how there are also those things in your partner which are not part of their true being; bits of unnecessary baggage they are carrying around, which are a hindrance. Reach out and bless your partner. Reach out your hands of healing and touch the parts of them that have not been integrated into their true being. Feel yourself loving them—all of them—the light and the dark places alike. Feel your power to embrace your partner, and the strength and affirmation your partner derives from your embrace. Feel how the sum of your power together is greater than either of you have as individuals. Sense your light shining more brightly as you come together: an increase of radiance. Thank the spirit of your partner for coming to be with you.

Now the two of you turn your attention outward, to become aware of another spirit. You notice that this spirit is different from the two of you. Its shining bubble of spirit is as large and as complex as your own. But the portion that represents the physical body is very small and unformed as yet. It is a spiritual giant in a tiny physical form. It is some distance away from you, and you beckon it closer. It moves toward you slowly. Do not try to pull it towards you any closer than it wishes to come. Let it find the distance between you which it is comfortable for it. It can stay at this distance while you become familiar with each other.

Notice the details of it. What colors are part of it? In what patterns do they move? What other characteristics does it have? Is it speaking to you? If so, what does it say? If it does not speak, do not try and force it. Just be there, fully present. Ask it what you can do for it in order to prepare for its incarnation. It may not respond with anything at all, or it may have a lengthy list of suggestions. Note carefully anything it tries to communicate, but do not pressure it to communicate.

Form your bubble of energy to a point that faces your fetus. Now make the point lengthen, like a strand of straight rope that goes out from you towards the spirit of the fetus. See this bright channel of energy reach your fetus, and join with its bubble of energy. Now feel energy flowing from you to the fetus. Let it feel your love and concern, your assurance that you want only what is best. Feel its energy flowing back along the path towards you. Receive that energy. Embrace it, make it one with you. Feel yourself enriched by this gift of light from another.

Then let the encounter draw to a close. As you are preparing to part, let the fetus decide if it wants to maintain the energy link, or to let it go for now, till the next time. If it wants to go, gently release your energy strand and let it blend back into you.

Thank the spirit of the fetus for coming to be with you, and sense it fade into the distance. Thank your partner for blending with you in this experience. Give your partner a final embrace, and allow them to fade away too. Become aware of how you are breathing; in and out, in and out, in and out. Feel your light form filling your physical form. Feel every part of your body filled with this radiant light. Appreciate each part of your physical body. When you are ready, open your eyes. Write down what you have just seen and felt. Write as many specifics as possible.

§   §   §

This meditation is a general introduction to the spirit of the baby, in which we just let the nature of the contact be whatever it will be. This exercise can be done several times, until you feel really comfortable being with the spirit of the child.

The purpose of the next exercise is to bring the level of communication from the general level to the specific. Once a pattern of communion is firmly established between the adults and the child, more specific information can be exchanged. It is rather like any human encounter; we need to feel comfortable in the presence of another human being before we begin to tell them our deepest secrets. We don't jump to deeper levels until we feel comfortable together. The above meditation is designed to set the stage in this way. Let the child set the pace. It may be very reluctant to come close at first; give it time to get used to your gestures of welcome. Don't try to force it.

Once the stage of familiarity is reached, then switch over to the following exercise. Before beginning, set up the room so you are comfortable, as you did before. Keep pen and paper handy, so that you can write down your observations at the end.

§ § §

FIFTH EXERCISE
RECEIVING ANGELIC WISDOM

Close your eyes. Breathe out, exhaling all the old, stale air from your lungs. Relax, and allow pure, clean, fresh air to be sucked back in. Breathe out and in, in this manner, several times. With each outbreath, feel the tension leave your body.

As you breathe in, feel the fresh air streaming over your brain and mind, washing out all the preoccupations in your head. Let all your concerns, your worries, fade into the background. Let the cool, white incoming air soothe your frustrations, smoothing over the rough patches in your life.

Visualize your body as being filled with green energy. This green energy is all the stored tensions that have been retained in your muscles and organs. See how this energy fills all of your limbs. Start at your feet. On each outbreath, feel the energy flowing out of your feet with the breath. Take as many outbreaths as required to clear out this green fluid from every nook and cranny of your feet.

Then go up your calves, thighs, pelvis, and work your way up. Allow the green energy to flow out of your shoulders on your breath, then clear your head and neck. Keep going till no tension or tightness remain. Feel how completely relaxed your body has become.

Now let your attention review each part of your body again, to see if there are still any remaining pockets of the tension-energy. Find the subtle places where tension still lingers and allow it to flow easily out of you on the current of your breath.

You are now an empty form, limp and flaccid. Behind you, you can sense the presence of your true being. It is a beautiful, shining presence. It is nothing but love for you. Once again its presence enfolds you, and you melt into it. In the bubble of its presence, you know that you are perfectly safe. You know that you have come home. It feels wonderful to be with your light-self again. It welcomes you into itself, and you feel free, safe and secure.

Feel how perfect this true you is, how beautiful. Feel how there is nothing in the bubble of energy that is this being that could possibly threaten you, disturb you or upset you. It is fully you. It is truly you. Look and see the appearance of this being that is you. Look at the gorgeous colors, the perfect shapes.

Spend as much time as you like just appreciating the wonder of this being. Notice details about its form, and how it flows. Has it changed at all since you were with it last? Is it more distinct? Are its colors brighter? Merge every part of your outer self with it in ecstatic union.

Now take time to look around you, around you two-who-have-merged-into-one. Notice the light-presence of your partner coming towards you. See your partner coming slowly towards you, till your light-forms are close to each other.

Notice how perfect your partner is. Has your partner changed at all since you saw them last?

Reach out and bless your partner. Reach out your hands of healing and touch the parts of their outer being that have not been integrated into their true being. Feel yourself loving them—all of them—light and dark places. Feel your power to embrace your partner, and the strength and affirmation your partner derives from your embrace. Feel how the sum of your power together is greater than either of you have as individuals. Sense your radiance increasing as you come together. Thank the spirit of your partner for coming to be with you.

Now the two of you turn your attention outward, to become aware of another spirit, the spirit of your baby. Its shining bubble of spirit is as large and as complex as your own. But the portion that represents the physical body is very small and unformed as yet. It is a spiritual giant and a physical pygmy. It is some distance away from you, and you beckon it closer. It moves toward you. Do not try to pull it towards you any closer than it wishes to come. Let it find the distance between you which it is comfortable for it. Is this distance different from the previous time you saw it?

Just be there, fully present. Note the details. Can you see any details you could not see before?

Form your bubble of energy to a point that faces your fetus. Now make the point lengthen, into a strand of energy that goes out from you towards the spirit of the fetus. See this bright channel of energy reach your fetus, and join with its bubble of energy. Now feel energy flowing from you to the fetus. Let it feel your love and concern, your assurance that you want only what is best.

Feel its energy flowing back along the path towards you. Receive that energy. Embrace it, make it one with you. Feel yourself enriched by this gift of light from another.

Ask the spirit of the fetus what it needs from you. Ask it specific questions, and give it time to reply. If it does not reply after a little while, move on to the next question. Ask it:

- *What do I and my partner need to eat that will serve the needs of your growing body?*

- *What sort of physical environment does my body need in order to nurture yours?*

- *What sort of mental environment must I maintain in order to nurture yours?*

- *What sort of emotional climate do I need to maintain in order to nurture yours?*

- *What physical habits do I have that obstruct your growth and function?*

- *What mental habits do I have that obstruct your growth and function?*

- *What emotional habits do I have that obstruct your growth and function?*

- *What habits in my relationship with my partner do I have that obstruct your coming into your own?*

- *What sorts of people would you like around you while you are an infant, and cannot speak to me?*

- *What sorts of people would you like around you when you are a child?*

- *What physical place would best serve your growth?*

- *What is your primary purpose in coming to Earth?*

- *What are some of your secondary purposes?*

- *How can I help you with those?*

- *What are some of my purposes?*

- *How can you help me with these?*

- *What is your name?*

- *Do you have any closely related souls incarnating around this same time?*

- *Are there any books you would like me to read?*

- *Are there any people you would like me to talk to?*

- *What style of birthing would you most prefer?*

- *Who would you like as a (midwife, nurse, doctor)?*

- *Which friends and relatives, if any, would you like at the birth?*

- *How can I minimize stress for you after birth?*

- *How can I minimize stress for myself after your birth?*

- *How can I minimize stress for my partner after your birth?*

- *What color room would you like as a baby?*

- *What else should I know before your birth?*

- *What is the most important thing you would like me to remember after your birth?*

- *What else would you like to tell me?*

Let the encounter draw to a close. As you are preparing to part, let the fetus decide if it wants to maintain the energy link, or to let it go for now, till the next time. If it wants to go, gently release your energy strand and let it blend back into you.

Thank the spirit of the fetus for coming to be with you, and sense it fade into the distance. Thank your partner for blending with you in this experience. Give your partner a final embrace, and allow them to fade away too.

Become aware of how you are breathing: in and out, in and out, in and out. Feel your light form filling your physical form. Feel every part of your body filled with this radiant light. Feel and appreciate each part of your physical body. Feel yourself affirmed and strengthened by this experience. Enjoy your new sense of connection with the fetus, and know that it will be with you all day. When you are ready, open your eyes. Write down as many specifics as possible.

§   §   §

Repeat this meditation in a day or two, using your own list of questions.

You may turn back to this exercise from time to time for answers, as different situations arise in your life and pregnancy. As your relationship with the spirit of the fetus grows, you may find yourself being able to ask it more and more specific questions.

You Are In Control

Don't hesitate to check the information you receive during these meditations against other sources. If your partner is doing these exercises with you, their experience is a valuable counterpoint on your own. Ideas you feel you're getting from the spirit of the baby should make sense to your mind and heart as well.

These exercises are not a substitute for our minds, and the intuition and sensing we feel from other sources. As multifaceted beings, we must honor the wisdom of all aspects of ourselves. These meditations may put us in touch with one aspect. But to go overboard in one aspect and ignore the others misses the fullness of ourselves.

Don't be uncritical of the information you receive in your meditation times. You are the one who is in control of the process. You are not abandoning responsibility to a being who is guiding you from another plane.

But once you accept your own spiritual identity, you are in position to receive information on that level from the spiritual identity of your fetus, and open up a world of awareness you might never gain from material sources. This information can help you prepare for the birth and life of your child in the most optimum way.

PART THREE

Flowing In
Radiance

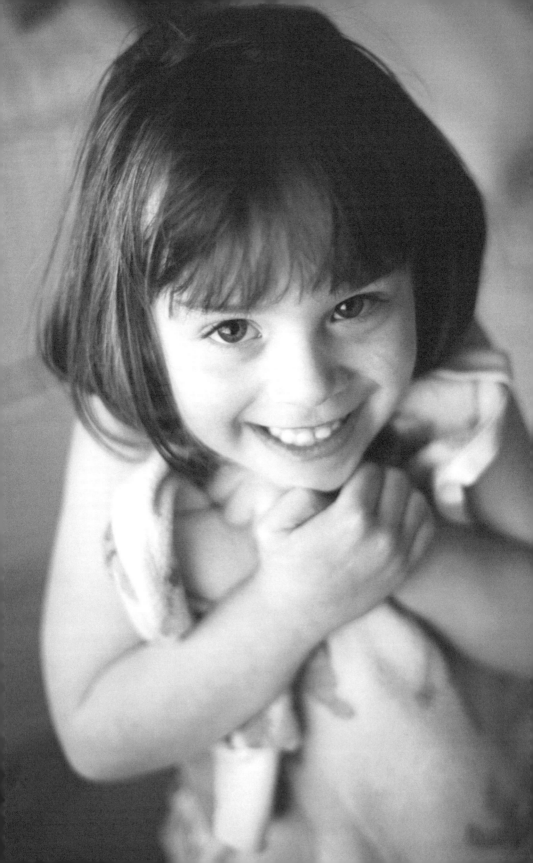

8

Radiance Exercises

O ur energy bodies are visible to some people, but invisible to most. They are sometimes described as a sphere extending two to five feet away from the physical body in all directions. The colors of this sphere differ from person to person, depending on the individual's characteristics. A person's field will change continuously, reflecting the general state of health, energy blockages, specific diseases, the emotional state, whether one is awake or asleep, and other factors.

When two people are together, their auras interact even when no physical contact takes place. Those who are more sensitive to auric qualities can consciously pick up information from the auras of others. Part of intuition is the ability to read the auric signals we are giving out all the time about our intentions, our general state and our specific qualities.

Within this bioenergy field that penetrates the physical body of each person, there are focus points for different kinds of energy, the chakras. Each chakra corresponds to a particular quality. There are seven chakras in traditional descriptive systems, nine in others, and twelve in a few.

On the physical level, the manifestation of these invisible bioenergetic points can be correlated with the endocrine system. There are seven endocrine glands. They are also referred to as the ductless glands, because, unlike sebaceous glands or salivary glands, their secretions do not flow through ducts to other parts of the body. The secretions of the endocrine glands pass directly into the bloodstream, and thus have an immediate effect on the entire body. The best known of the endocrine glands is the adrenal. When our adrenal glands are stimulated into the secretion of adrenaline, the "fight or flight" mechanism readies the whole body in seconds to respond to the exigencies of an emergency situation.

Endocrine Glands & Bioenergy Points

Because of this correlation between the bioenergetic and physical systems, many therapeutic effects can be obtained by treating the bioenergetic body, without intruding on the physical body. You don't need to touch the physical body in order to affect it. The invisible levels of wellness are interconnected with physical wellness.

With practice, it is possible to develop our awareness of these invisible levels of being. As we raise our sensitivity to this whole field of function, our invisible senses become more and more acute, and we see more of what is happening in these areas. We rely less on what we can see, smell, hear, touch and taste and more on what we "sense without senses" to construct our picture of the world and of other people.

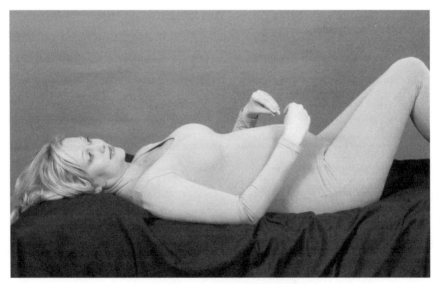

Specific Pattern – Mother Only

Utilizing this area of perception, we can interact with the unborn child, connecting in a powerful, radiant way on a spiritual level. The exer-

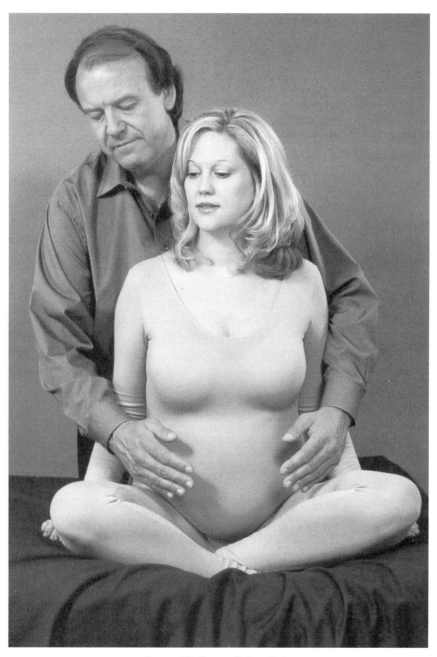

General Pattern – Father Only

cise below can be done with a child in utero, a newborn, or an older child. It is easier if the child is asleep.

§ § §

SIXTH EXERCISE
DIVINE ENERGY CONNECTION

Make yourself comfortable in a quiet room that is not too bright. Become aware of your breathing. Breathe slowly in and out, allowing all the concerns of the day to exit on your outbreaths. Feel your mind becoming quiet as you focus on your breath. Feel your heart becoming still, as all the things that have disturbed it flow out of your body on your breath. Keep focusing on your breathing, in and out, until your body, mind and heart are all perfectly still.

Visualize a beam of light coming down from above to rest on your head. This beam is white, shining, pure, and bathes you with a gentle radiance. Imagine the source of the light. The light is coming from the Lord of light, the Supreme Being of love, the One who cares intimately for the well-being of this planet. Whatever your highest vision of Godhead is, imagine the light proceeding from this One to touch the top of your head. Feel your responsiveness to this infinite sea of love. Your thankfulness ascends back up the light beam. Now visualize the beam of light flowing over your body and down your arms to your hands. As it flows over your hands, hold your hands in such a way as to focus this energy, as though you were pointing it, using all four fingers and your thumb.

See the shining essence of your partner coming towards you. Direct the stream of energy you create with your hands toward the energy field of your partner. As the energy touches them, the colors and intensity of their energy field intensify. Keep your energy beam tightly focused, using your fingers as a pointer. As you bathe them in this radiance, feel how they respond to your invisible touch.

Now open your hands so that the energy is more diffused. Hold them about a foot to eighteen inches away from the baby. Gently allow this diffused energy to make contact with the baby's energy field. Keep a stable radiance coming from your hands, and feel the intensification of your own field and that of the baby.

Allow the intensity of the love radiance pouring from your hands to increase. Let the pressure build, but to a point at which it is still comfortable to the child. Allow the current coming from you to increase, and an intensified response to reciprocate from the child.

Hold this current of love steady. Keep in mind that you are not the originator of this stream of love, but the transmitter. Remain totally responsive to the One above whose energy you are focusing. Keep your mind centered in the beam of love coming to you from above.

You may feel certain patterns in the energy field of the baby shift. Don't try too hard to figure out what they are, for this will take your mind off of its connection to the One above. Whatever you feel happening, stay connected upwards. Do not let your mind stray. Keep your response flowing upward towards the Supreme One even as the light streams from your hands to the baby.

After a certain amount of time, you may feel that the pattern of radiance is complete. When this occurs, allow the intensity of the energy coming from your hands to taper off gently. Move your hands further from the child. Move slowly, being careful to keep the connection with the baby.

Turn your hands so that the palms point upward. Let your thanks flow upward to God for the privilege of transmitting and sharing His energy.

When you have given thanks, turn your palms inward and place your hands on your heart. Feel how still your heart and mind are, and how full. Remember this feeling whenever you see your hand today. Remember it throughout the whole day, especially when you are distracted, or when events come up to pull your emotions off center.

Feel your breathing once more. Experience the air flowing gently in and out. Feel how refreshed and new you feel. Give thanks for this experience, and open your eyes when you are ready.

§ § §

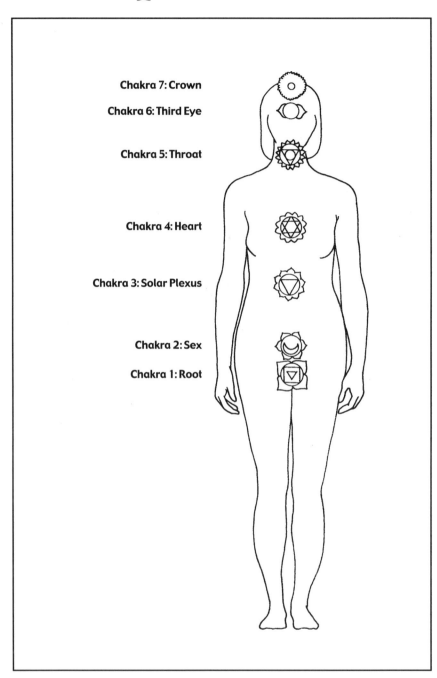

Chakra 7: Crown

Chakra 6: Third Eye

Chakra 5: Throat

Chakra 4: Heart

Chakra 3: Solar Plexus

Chakra 2: Sex

Chakra 1: Root

Chakras

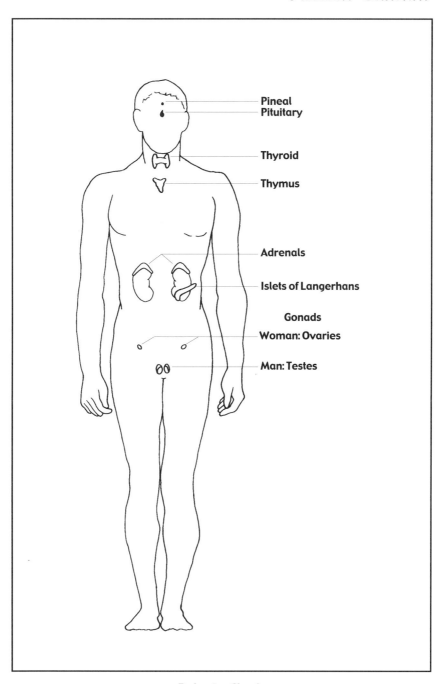

Pineal
Pituitary

Thyroid

Thymus

Adrenals

Islets of Langerhans

Gonads
Woman: Ovaries

Man: Testes

Endocrine Glands

Maintaining Upward Orientation

During this exercise it is important to keep your own patterns of consciousness clear. The more intense the experience, the more likely that your mind and heart will become stirred up. Strong spiritual experiences may jar loose various excited thought patterns. If you take your attention away from the moment in order to explore some attractive thought that pops up out of the subconscious, you will remove yourself from the present moment and what is really happening.

The purpose of this exercise is not to generate fodder for the mind. You are working with extremely sensitive and delicate areas of your baby's well-being. It is crucial to remain centered while engaging in this type of work. This is done by remaining focused on your connection with God, and not allowing your attention to be distracted from God by what is happening around you or within you—especially within you. The life stream must be held steady, by a mind and heart that are totally focused on being a conduit for spirit from above.

If you discover you do not have the ability to do this, you can contact an Emissary attunement server at www.emissaries.org. Attunement servers have many years of experience in maintaining this upward connection as the life stream is focused. Or you can book an attunement with me through www.SoulHealings.com; distance doesn't matter! The guidance of an experienced person is highly recommended during this delicate and lovely process of connecting parents and child.

Forming Radiant Habits

If you are doing this exercise with a young child that's asleep, you may observe the child's body moving during the course of the exercise. You may notice rapid eye movements, or limb movements, or settling in and getting comfortable, or even signs of discomfort. These effects are common and normal. Spiritual power may produce strong physical effects. Whatever experience the child is having may be heightened by such a process.

Once you are practiced in the art of focusing this divine radiance, you will discover that you begin to do it instinctively. You no longer react to crises by becoming upset, frustrated or angry. Instead, you regard crises as opportunities to send out this spiritual radiance to the individuals involved, or to your own disturbed mind and heart. You instinctively adopt a radiant stance whenever the road gets rocky. Spirit becomes your primary resource for dealing with any situation.

The Seventh Exercise below puts you in touch with all the specific contact points in the child's body into which you can direct the radiance of love.

Spirit Creates Form

Each endocrine gland has a corresponding spirit. The spirit is the divine quality with which that part of the body is associated. When we direct radiance to a particular part of the body, we are not primarily working with the physical organ. We are interested in effecting change on the spiritual level that underlies and affects the physical.

Spirit underlies form. As we do our appropriate work on the spiritual level, the physical levels of things fall into place. There is no need for us to try and manipulate physical form to produce healing. As the spirit is pure and true, the form will reflect it. So although we use the endocrine glands as contact points, we are not doing these exercises for the benefit of the glands. We are doing it for the benefit of the whole, and wholeness is found in spirit.

Spirit is not an undifferentiated mass, as you will know from the above exercise. It has particular characteristics. Around these spiritual vortices, physical form takes shape. The purpose of the exercises is to promote an effective connection between spirit and form.

Disease results from a blockage of the connection between spirit and form. The goal of these exercises is not to effect any particular change in form. It is to allow a free flow of spirit to form, with the understanding that when it is allowed free access, spirit will make whatever changes are required in form.

There are certain spiritual poles around which physical matter is organized. Each primary radiation point in the physical body, each endocrine gland, has a particular spirit with which it is associated. The following chart lists these correlations.

GLAND:	SPIRIT:
Pineal	Love
Pituitary	Womb
Thyroid	Life
Thymus	Purity
Islets of Langerhans	Blessing
Adrenals	Purpose
Gonads	Earth

As we move though each one, you will become sensitive to each spirit, and the effect that spirit (and the absence of it) has on physical form. You will nurture each of these aspects in the child, and encourage an optimal transfer of energy between the spirit of the child and his or her form.

Methods

The following exercise will familiarize you with these contact points in the baby. You can do this exercise with a child in utero, after birth, at any subsequent age, or with your partner as the subject. If your children have reached the squirmy stage, it is most convenient to do it while they are asleep.

If both partners wish to participate in doing this with the child as the subject, one partner should do the Sixth Exercise (above), holding a gen-

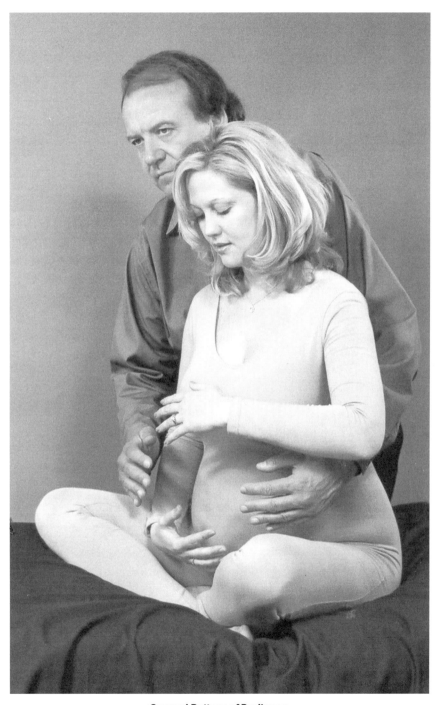

General Pattern of Radiance

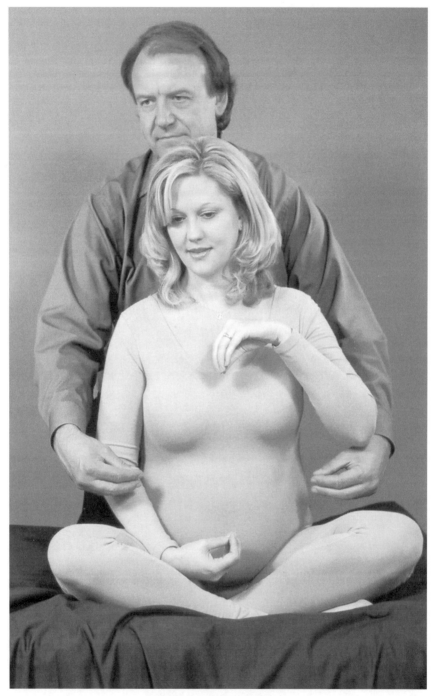

Specific Patterns of Radiance

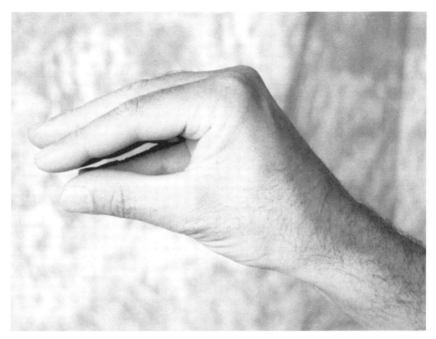

Hand Position A: Strong Focus

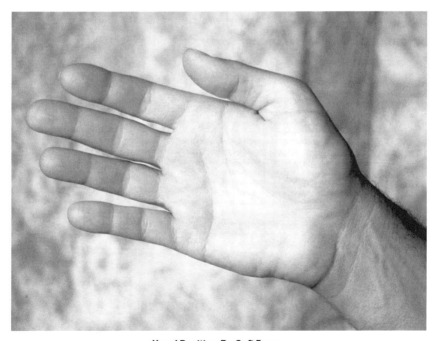

Hand Position B: Soft Focus

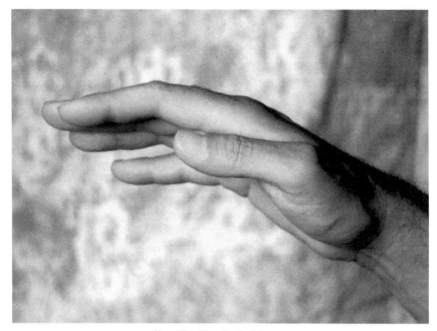

Hand Position B: Soft Focus

eral pattern of radiance, while the other does the Seventh Exercise (below), which involves a specific pattern. The parent holding the general pattern is setting up an atmosphere of blessing around the entire circumference of the baby's bioenergy field, while the parent holding the specific pattern is focusing energy on specific bioenergy points. The photographs in this chapter demonstrate these positions.

It is also possible for one parent to channel radiance to the child using the contact points on the other parent. One parent does it with the other as subject, while they both maintain a clear mental image of the child.

For a mother doing this exercise alone, with her child in utero as the subject, hand positions A and B may also be used. See the chart and illustrations below for details.

Before you begin the exercise below, put yourself in a physical environment that is still, and free of distractions. A darkened room may be helpful, with just a little light present. Play, at very low volume, some soothing music. You can have a friend or your partner read you the

Meditation, or you can record it and play it back. If you have downloaded the audio version of this book, use that.

If two partners are each doing one of the two exercises, both should do the same things during Part One, the first ten paragraphs, of the Seventh Exercise below.

After that, one continues with the specific hand movements of the Seventh Exercise while the other simply holds their hands in a general pattern of radiance as described in the Sixth Exercise. Review the endocrine diagram at the beginning of this chapter before commencing this Exercise, to refresh yourself on the location of each gland. You may want to keep the book open to that page, so that you can glance at the reference points occasionally.

§ § §

SEVENTH EXERCISE
RADIANCE PREPARATION
PART ONE

Close your eyes. Breathe out, exhaling all the old, stale air from your lungs. Relax, and allow pure, clean, fresh air to be sucked back in. Breathe out and in in this manner several times. With each outbreath, feel the tension leave your body. As you breathe in, feel the fresh air streaming over your brain and mind, washing out all the thoughts in your head. Let all your concerns, your worries, fade into the background. Let the cool, white incoming air soothe your frustrations, smoothing over the rough patches in your life.

Visualize your body as being filled with green energy. This green energy is all the stored tensions that have been retained in your muscles and organs. Picture this energy filling all of your limbs. Start at your feet. On each outbreath, feel the energy flowing out of your feet with the breath. Take as many outbreaths as required to clear out this green fluid from every nook and cranny of your feet.

Then go up your calves, thighs, pelvis, and work your way up. Spend enough time on each place to allow all the green tension energy to flow out of you completely. When you have completely cleared your shoulders of this fluid green energy, and each part

95

of your body feels completely limp, see the energy that fills your head. Start at the back of your skull, and begin to expel it with each breath. Keep going till even the smallest cavities in your head have been emptied of the green energy, and no tension or tightness remain.

Finally, empty your neck and mouth of the fluid, and feel how completely relaxed your body has become.

Now let your attention review each part of your body again, to see if there are still any remaining pockets of the tension-energy. Find the subtle places where tension is still lingering, and allow it to flow easily out of you on the current of your breath.

You are now an empty form, limp and flaccid. Behind you, though, you can sense the presence of another being. This other being is a beautiful, shining presence. It is nothing but love for you. Its presence enfolds you, and you melt into it. In the bubble of its presence, you know that you are perfectly safe. In its presence you are at home. It welcomes you into itself, and your heart can rest in the knowledge that you have come home. You are free, safe and secure. You feel an upsurge of thankfulness that you have contacted this being, who is your true self, once again.

Feel how perfect this being is, how beautiful. Feel how there is nothing in the bubble of energy that is this being that could possibly threaten you, disturb you or upset you. It is fully you. It is truly you. Look and see the appearance of this being that is you. Look at the gorgeous colors, the perfect shapes. Spend as much time as you would like just appreciating the wonder of this being. Notice details about its form, and how it flows. Merge every part of yourself with it in ecstatic union.

Visualize a beam of light coming down from above to rest on your head. This beam is white, shining, pure, and bathes you with a gentle radiance. Imagine the source of the light. The light is coming from the Lord of light, the supreme being of love, the One who has ultimate responsibility for the coordination of this world. Whatever your highest vision of godhead is, imagine the light proceeding from this One to touch the top of your head. Feel your responsiveness to this infinite sea of love. Feel your thankfulness ascending back up the light beam.

Now visualize the beam of light flowing over your body and down your arms to your hands. As it flows over your hands, hold your hands in such a way as to focus this energy, as though you were pointing it, using all four fingers and your thumb (Hand Position A). Direct the stream of energy you create in this way towards the energy field of your child. As the energy touches the child, the colors and intensity of their energy field intensify. Keep your energy beam tightly focused using your fingers as a pointer. As you bathe them in this radiance, feel how they respond to your invisible touch.

Now open your hands so that the energy is more diffused (Hand Position B). Hold them about a foot to eighteen inches away from the baby. Keep a stable radiance coming from your hands, and feel the intensification of your own field and that of the baby. Notice the details of it. What colors are part of it? In what patterns do they move? What other characteristics does it have? Has it changed since you sensed it last?

§ § §

PART TWO

Once you have felt the general energy field of the baby, and directed your radiance towards it using your flat hands, point your fingers to focus the energy more precisely. (Hand Position A). From a general glow around your hands, the energy becomes a focused beam.

Direct this beam to a point at the junction of the child's head and torso. The head represents the heavenly place of control, and the torso represents the earthly place of response. As you are doing this, hold a strong image of your child always responding to the creative currents that come from Heaven in every moment. Feel any blockages that impede this current dissolving, so that the current of heavenly intent flows freely from Heaven, the realm of control, into the Earth, the realm of response. Imagine your child always balanced at this crossover point, joining Heaven and Earth in the divine union of creative energies. (Radiance Meditation One).

Once you sense that this pattern of right action is established in the fetus, you will feel that this point of radiance is complete and it is time to move on.

Move your hands, focusing them on a point in the center of the top of the child's head. Become aware of the connection point on the top of your own head with the silver cord coming down from

Heaven. Feel the energy pouring from your hands connecting with that same point on the top of the child's head. Picture the silver cord that comes from the top of the child's head going up into Heaven. As the energy radiates from your hands, see that heavenly connection strengthening. See the child's cord pulsating with the energy coming down from above. Feel the love that is pouring in to the child from this connection with spirit (Radiance Meditation Two).

Spend a few minutes just rejoicing in this flow. Enjoy it. Then, when the flow is steady, unwavering, firmly established, move on to the next contact point.

The next contact point is just below the first, moving from the top of the child's head down the body. It is the pituitary gland. It represents the Spirit of the Womb. It is so close to the pineal that you hardly have to move your hands to touch it. Cradle the Spirit of the Womb in your hands. Feel this spirit grow strong as you pour your spirit out upon it. Feel the energy moving though your hands to energize this part of the child. As the radiant current intensifies, feel your own pituitary gland start to glow. The Spirit of the Womb is a symbol of the place where Truth dwells. Truth is the control point for the rest of the body. As you touch this gland you extend your radiant influence to all the other glands and systems (Radiance Meditation Three).

Spend a few minutes just rejoicing in this contact. Then, when the contact is steady, unwavering, firmly established, gently move on to the next contact point.

The thyroid gland represents the Spirit of Life. As you move your hand down to make connection with this spirit, imagine your child glowing with life. Imagine the child's whole experience to be vibrant, rich, confident. Become aware of your breathing once again. Breathe the breath of life into the child's third chakra. With each breath you let out, visualize breathing out a gentle, pale blue fluid into your child's throat. Picture this blue fluid bestowing on your child a full life, a wonderful life (Radiance Meditation Four).

When you have a steady pattern of connection with the thyroid, move on to the next point.

The thymus gland represents the Spirit of Purification. As you move your hand down to make contact with this point, see your child being cleansed of all the impurities that will go through them. See them easily processing all the negative energy that they

*receive. It passes easily through their system, not affecting them.
Any poison that they ingest, physically, emotionally or mentally,
passes easily through them, as their filtration system has no trouble
in handling it. As they pass through the world on their journey,
they are able to purify the Earth by their passage (Radiance
Meditation Five).*

*When you sense that the child's purification system is working
properly, enjoy the perfection of it for a few moments, then go on to
the next contact point.*

*The Islets of Langerhans represent the Spirit of Blessing. See
your child blessing people as a pattern in their life. See the life of
your child being a blessing to God. Imagine your child as a radiant being whose every step through the Earth brings blessing to all
they touch. See God being pleased with the child.*

*Imagine your child's hand touching the hands of all the people
they will ever meet, and those hands being blessed by the touch of
this blessed hand. Envision your child being ingenious in finding
ways to bless people that no one else can touch. See your child's
capacity to bless growing strong as you radiate energy to it from
your hands (Radiance Meditation Six).*

*When the pattern of blessing is strong and stable in your child,
move your hands down to the next contact point.*

*The Spirit of Purpose is represented in the human body by the
adrenal glands. See your child as having singleness of purpose. This
child's single purpose will be to serve God. Don't try and place any
strong specific image on what this might mean. The child will find
its own way of serving God. But the spirit of singleness of purpose
means that the child will always have its eyes fixed on the most
important thing in life: the connection upwards to God.*

*The child may live in the world, but it will always have its
vision trained on the divine. Its eyes will be unwaveringly fixed on
its divine purpose; it will remain undistracted by lesser purposes.
With a fixity of purpose, it will prosper in all that it does. It will
see God in everything. It will lead a magical life, full of wonder.
With its purpose fixed in God, all else will fall into place.
Everything else will work for this baby, if this focus of spirit is there
(Radiance Meditation Seven).*

*Celebrate with your child, through the radiance of your hands,
the Spirit of Singleness of Purpose. When you sense that this pattern*

of obedience is firm and unwavering in the child, move your hands downward to the next contact point.

The Gonads or sexual glands represent the Spirit of the New Earth. As you allow radiance to pour through your hands directed at this point on the baby's body, fill your mind with the Spirit of the New Earth. The New Earth is what is created when the New Heaven is in place.

When your baby's spiritual orientation is steadfast, centered in the New Heaven, all the forms that this child requires for creation on the Earth plane, the New Earth, will be there. We sense so strongly in this moment that the spirit of things underlies the form of things. This baby will be finely attuned to spirit. With this orientation, the form of things will fall into place automatically.

Picture your baby creating things effortlessly on the Earth plane because the spirit plane is the primary reality for them. They are not responsive to the Earth; they are responsive to Heaven, and as a result, Heaven floods down to manifest through them into the Earth. As this happens through your baby, the Earth is made new. It rejoices to be renewed, remade, blessed and recreated by the presence upon it of God-centered human beings. Your baby will renew the Earth, as it lives in Heaven (Radiance Meditation Eight).

Once you feel a strong connection made with the Spirit of the New Earth through the Gonads of your baby, enjoy feeling the energy of it for a few moments.

Once you are done with radiation to the gonads, move your hands back up the baby's body to the point where you started: the neck area, between head and torso. Feel the current of connection between the Spirit of Heaven and the Spirit of Earth, moving through this point on the baby's body. This current may feel measurably stronger now than when you began, or it may feel the same. Either way is fine. Celebrate for a few minutes the power of life moving down from Heaven into manifestation in the Earth through the body of your child (Radiance Meditation Twelve).

Now move your hands gently upwards as though you were cradling the top of the baby's head. Let your hands move from a point of strong focus (Hand Position A) to a point of soft focus (Hand Position B). Imagine you are cradling the baby's mind.

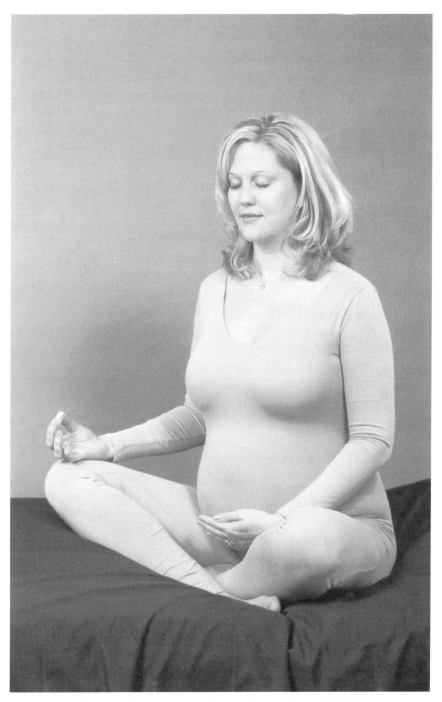

Personal Meditation, with Energy Flowing Through Child

Picture the thoughts that are filling their mind at this moment being full of creativity and peace.

Visualize this child blessing everyone they come into contact with their whole life long, through the thoughts that pass through their brain. Picture their conscious mind being able to easily give articulation to the beauty that lives within them. Picture their words and thoughts moving out to thousands of people during their lifetime, bringing healing to everyone they ever think about or talk to (Radiance Meditation Nine).

Once you have spent some time surrounding the baby's head in this way, move your hands again. One hand should be on either side of the cord that connects the baby to Heaven above. Keeping your hands open, let your palms face away from the baby and towards Heaven. Give thanks for the experience you have just had. Give thanks for the miracle of being able to connect consciously with your baby.

Give this child that you have been given back to Heaven as a gift. Know that it is not your child, but Heaven's child. This child is Heaven's way of blessing the Earth. This child is the mechanism by which the Spirit of Heaven may touch the Spirit of Earth. Present the child as a living offering to Heaven.

Give thanks for the privilege you have just had of conducting the Spirits of Heaven down into the child, through the medium of your own capacities of heart, mind, body and spirit. Feel how refreshed these capacities are by their channeling of the divine into human form. Become aware of how you are breathing; in and out, in and out, in and out. Feel your light form filling your physical form. Feel every part of your body filled with this radiant light. Feel and appreciate each part of your physical body. When you are ready, open your eyes.

§ § §

If you find your attention wanders during this Exercise, or you are unable to accommodate the intensity of it at times, remember to keep breathing rhythmically. Your breathing will always help to connect you with the physical plane.

You can also do this Exercise in another way: Instead of directing both hands towards the infant using Hand Position A, keep one hand facing palm upward during the entire process (Hand Position B). This will connect you even more strongly upwards to spirit, and will prevent you from losing sight of the spiritual connection which is the purpose of the Exercise.

You may find that one hand has a dominant role in the radiation process. In this case, visualize the current flowing out of this hand and into the baby, through the baby and back into the other hand, after which it flows upwards to Heaven.

The hand that is dominant while offering radiance will not necessarily be the one that is dominant in earthly tasks. You may be left handed as a rule, yet feel that your right hand is dominant when allowing energy to flow through.

Alternately, you may sense that one hand is dominant during one phase of the process, but when you move on to another stage of meditation, dominance shifts to the other hand. Your sensitivity to the currents of spirit increases with practice, and you will become easily aware of these subtle energy differences.

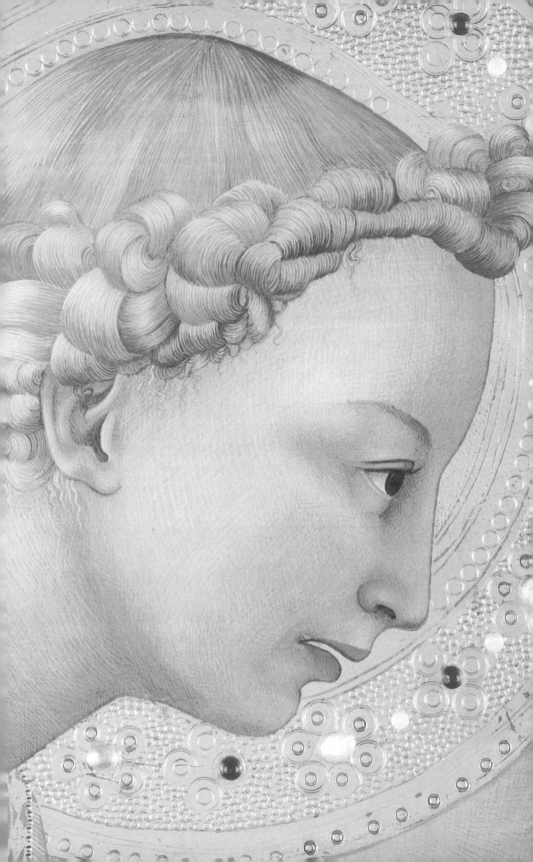

9

Radiance to the Pineal
The Spirit of the Crown

The uppermost chakra is commonly referred to as the crown chakra. Correlations have been made between the crown chakra and the haloes often depicted around the heads of holy figures in ancient art. The crown chakra is often represented as a golden globe of light above the head.

The physical point of correlation for the crown chakra is the pineal gland. This is a small ductless gland in the center of the cranial cavity, between the left and right lobe of the brain, whose functions remain obscure to science.

The spirit associated with the pineal body is the Spirit of Love. The Spirit of Love is the supreme spirit, from which all else proceeds. The Spirit of Love embodies all the Spirits below it. It is the primary connection with the divine. While this point is connected upwards, our physical body has life. When this connection is severed, it dies. The pineal represents the transcendence point at which the unmanifest realm of spirit first becomes manifest as form.

The exercises in this book that link specific divine qualities to a general spiritual connection are of a different order, and are therefore called Radiance Meditations. A Radiance Meditation is a conscious invocation of the spirit associated with a particular physical point. In subsequent chapters we will begin to consider how to direct the flow of the life current into each of the seven primary physical contact points. You will use one of the exercises in Chapter Eight (Sixth Exercise) to connect with the spirit of the fetus, then follow it with the Radiance Meditation for that chapter. To recap:

- Complete Sixth Exercise
- Go from there to Radiance Meditation in the chapter you are working with.

The Sixth Exercise in Chapter Eight works with any or all of the Radiance Meditations found in subsequent chapters.

Radiance Meditation One starts with the joint between head and neck, the crossover point, where the atlas and axis vertebrae allow the human body to perform the astonishing feat of moving the head both up and down and side-to-side. For this meditation, position your hands at the top of the spine, at the base of the skull, on either side of the head.

Radiance Meditation Two picks up with the pineal gland. Move right into this meditation after you're done with Radiance Meditation One. Then move on, point by point, from there. For convenience, each point you will visit after Radiance Meditation Two is a separate brief chapter, beginning with Chapter Ten.

§ § §

RADIANCE MEDITATION ONE
THE CROSSOVER POINT
THE JUNCTION OF HEAVEN AND EARTH

Become aware of your breathing. Slow each breath to the point where you are conscious of every part of the path the air travels in and out of you. Become so attuned to the energy of your breath that you can sense every molecule as it passes in and out of your system. With each inbreath sense your connection to spirit. Draw the energy of your divine truth in with each inbreath. Center your mind, your thoughts, your whole attention on radiant love.

As you breathe out, feel your personal presence grow stronger. With each outbreath feel the potency of your spiritual presence increase. Feel the strength of radiance which you reflect intensify. Become fully and powerfully you.

Focus the energy moving through you by pointing your hands (Hand Position A). Place your hands on either side of the point represented by the top of the baby's neck. This is the location of the Atlas and Axis vertebrae, upon which the head pivots on top of the spinal column. Feel the energy pour from your hands into this area.

This point represents the junction between Heaven and Earth. Heaven is the realm of control, symbolized here by the head. The Earth is the place of response, response to the will and patterns originating in Heaven. It is represented by the torso. When this crossover point is clear of obstructions and functioning properly, the essences of Heaven pour through it into the Earth.

Visualize this crossover point being a clear unobstructed channel for the spiritual essences of your baby to move into form. Allow the love that pours from your fingers to gently dissolve any blockages in this channel. Sense the divine energy moving clearly and freely through this pathway and into the physical form. Hold your hands over this point in the same position until you sense that there is a clear and unobstructed flow through this point. The flow should be continuous and stable before you move on.

When you sense that this flow is consistent, move your hands gently to a point that represents the top of the baby's head. Keep your hand movement smooth, being very conscious that you are touching the sacred spiritual body of another being.

§   §   §

RADIANCE MEDITATION TWO
THE SPIRIT OF LOVE: THE PINEAL GLAND

Move your hands slightly in the general area of the baby's head until you sense, using your spiritual eyes, that you have made firm contact with the baby's pineal. Picture a stream of light pouring from your hands into the gland. It is a laser-like, brilliant white beam of love. It stimulates the area and cements the connection with the stream of God's love coming into the baby's head from above.

107

See the stream of vibrant energy that pours down from Heaven through the top of the baby's head, connecting the child to God. Caress this beam of light. Love the connection that this beam makes between the divine all, the Tao, and the earthly form. Cradle this energy beam in your hands as you celebrate its connection with the physical contact point available in the pineal.

Feel these intentions move through you into the child. Speak the words aloud if you feel moved to do so:

"You are love. Love underlies every other aspect of your functioning. Love is the essence of your nature. Love is what you live for. It is this constant love stream coming from God that sustains your physical life. If this silver cord were not present, your physical form would cease to be alive. This column of love-substance penetrates your whole body and every part of it. It penetrates every other endocrine gland and energy point below it. It is the supreme principle of the universe, to which all else must be connected to survive. Always refer everything else in your whole life back to love, my dearest one. This is your constant reference point.

"In this moment I join my love to your love, allowing our columns of love to blend. They become more intense as they reinforce each other. In this moment I affirm my connection with the Divine. It is only because of my connection with the divine that I have anything to offer you. Affirming the solidity of my own spiritual centering allows me to direct and focus this current of love coming to you. Know, my child, that this love does not come from me in a personal sense. It is given freely by God, and as I open my heart and receive it into myself, it is mine to give freely.

"You will never be short of love. There is no scarcity of love. You do not have to hoard love, or be afraid that if you love certain people you will not have enough left over for others. You cannot claim love or possess love. You can only give love. As it is given, it overflows in the heart of the giver. God is love. God is infinite. Therefore love is infinite. I celebrate in this moment your connection with God in love."

§ § §

Once you sense that the flow of love is as fully received as it can possibly be by the baby's form, slowly move your hands to the next contact point: the Pituitary, which represents the Spirit of the Womb. The Meditation concepts for the Pituitary are found in the next chapter, Chapter Ten.

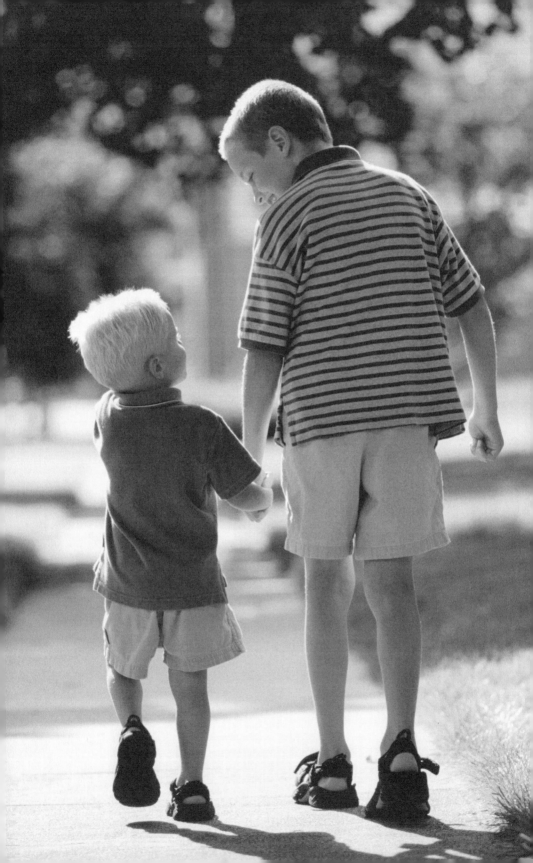

10

Radiance to the Pituitary
The Spirit of the Womb

The physical womb is the place in which life is created. As you are able to create the vibrational space in which spiritual life may grow—the spiritual womb—blessings will be born forth into your experience. The womb in which spiritual life is born is the Womb of Truth. In the Womb of Truth, the seed of Love is fertilized. The product of their union is sacred Life.

Check the location of the pituitary gland on the chart in Chapter Eight before beginning this exercise. The pituitary is sometimes referred to as the master gland, since the hormones it secretes affect the secretion of hormones by other glands. The purpose of Radiance Meditation Three is to allow you to picture the control that this master gland exerts being true to the directives of the child's soul throughout the child's life.

§ § §

RADIANCE MEDITATION THREE
THE SPIRIT OF TRUTH: THE PITUITARY

Be aware of how deeply relaxed your body is. Breathe deeply. With each inbreath, breathe in a shining white radiance. With every outbreath, feel yourself coming more and more to focus. Feel this energy that you channel becoming more and more focused, more and more intense.

Move your hands to a point that represents the center of the baby's head. Use your spiritual eyes to sense where the pituitary is located. Feel a steady stream of radiance emerge from your finger-tips and into the pituitary. Allow your mind to be flooded with the Spirit of the Womb. Be acutely conscious of the atmosphere of nurturing, safety and protection that you are creating.

Picture your baby developing in a manner that is utterly true to the inner reality. Let there be no deviance from the perfect focus of truth in any way.

With the Spirit of the Womb of Truth filling your mind, allow the current of truth moving under the dominion of the Spirit of Love through your hands to increase. Allow the current of truth to intensify. With every breath you breathe out, breathe the spirit of truth into the baby's heart and mind. Allow this master gland in your own brain to move into the Spirit of perfect Truth. Keep it there unwavering. Feel the infinite love coming down from above igniting all truth in your heart and filling your understanding with discernment of truth. Hold yourself steadfast in the current of God's truth flowing out of Heaven in each moment.

Visualize a radiant line of connection drawn between this focus point of truth in your own brain and the brain of your baby. As you become steadfast in truth, so the child cannot be other than steadfast in truth. As you make room in your consciousness for nothing other than truth, harboring no deceit, no lies, no deception, no double-mindedness, the radiance of sanctity will surround even your physical form. The truth of love will uplift and bless every part of your emotional, mental and physical world.

As you recognize your own sacredness, your child will see God in the flesh. As your form becomes God's temple, the child will always have a place to worship. As your experience becomes the womb in which the Spirit of Truth always dwells, the child will grow up in safety. The Womb of Truth is the most precious gift you can give in which to nurture your baby.

Once this spirit has come to full radiant focus through your fingers pointed toward the pituitary gland of the child, become aware of your inbreath and your outbreath. You are breathing in the love of God and breathing out His truth as it is expressed through your form.

§ § §

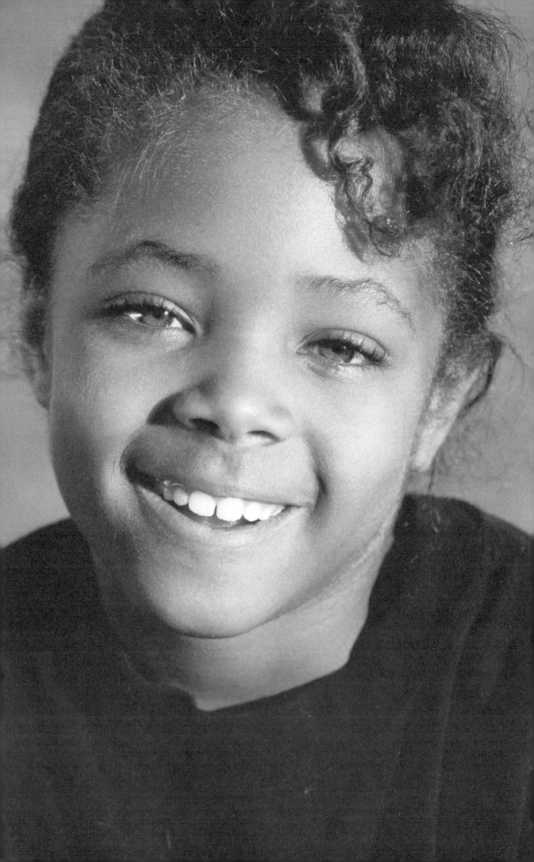

11

Radiance to the Thyroid
The Spirit of Life

The thyroid gland is located close to the Adam's apple—the bulge in the center of the throat. Refer to the illustration in Chapter Eight if you need to make sure you know where to find the thyroid.

As well as regulating the body's metabolic rate, the thyroid gland secretes a hormone essential to physical growth. This is merely the physical manifestation of the spiritual focus of the thyroid: to provide a physical contact point for the expression of the Spirit of Life into the body.

The thyroid is the physical focus of the Spirit of Life. This spirit follows Love and Truth, since Life is born after gestation in the sacred Womb of Truth.

Life is a force that bursts forth irresistibly when the Womb of Truth is exposed to the steady stream of the current of Love. Life does not have to be engendered or deliberately created. It is like the spark that is given off when a positive and negative pole touch each other. The spark does not have to be created in and of itself; it is a sure consequence of the interaction of positive and negative currents.

In the same way, Life bursts forth automatically when Love and Truth are in place. Life is irrepressible. In the springtime, unable to contain herself any longer, nature bursts forth with an incredible proliferation and profusion of fresh, shining forms. Nature's innate desire to create can, at a certain point, no longer be suppressed by winter, and bursts forth to transform the whole world. In the same way, when the Father of Love and the Mother of Truth are honored, the Child of Life cannot help but be born.

Your baby is a sacred representation of this principle at work. The life in the body of this child does not need to be created by our conscious minds. There is little we can do to encourage the growth of the physical form of this child. We need simply to step back and let life have its way. If life is allowed to have its way, it is perfectly capable of organizing complex molecules to build millions of cells and create a baby. It does not need an instruction book to do this. Ordered creativity is inherent to life. Life orders and organizes, and when we allow an increase of life in our personal experience it brings with it the gifts of purpose, ease and organic organization.

We create a dynamic bond of life between ourselves and the child by communing with the Spirit of Life shaping our child through the thyroid.

§ § §

RADIANCE MEDITATION FOUR
THE SPIRIT OF LIFE: THE THYROID

Move your hands down the child's body to the front of the throat. With pointed fingers directing the flow of energy, make contact with this point. Use your sensing of the invisible currents of spirit to direct you accurately to this location.

As your hands direct love into the area of your baby's body which represents the thyroid gland, picture this infant bursting with life, with vigor, with joy, with the irrepressible exuberance of new life. Picture life as a glittering stream of energy surrounding the entire planet and permeating all its creatures. The amount of this sacred life-energy which we allow into our bodies determines how full our experience of life will be.

Picture this life energy flowing through the child's body without obstruction. Now picture the quantity of this life-energy increasing. Feel the pace of life within the child quicken, as the life-energy pouring through your focused hands intensifies. Feel the potential that this brings.

As this increased flow of the life current passes through the child's body, it nurtures and sustains the child; it enriches the child's experience. Rather than a miserable restricted trickle of life passing though the child, picture a gushing stream of life substance flowing though the child's body. Allow your focused hands to facilitate the increase of this flow. As you send these sparkling granules of life-energy coursing through the child's body, imagine them coursing more and more strongly through your own body too.

You cannot give what you do not have. Only as you allow an increased expression of the life current though your own experience will you be able to share with the child with this immeasurable gift of life. Imagine your own body filled to capacity with these flowing, brilliant granules. Imagine the pleasure God has in seeing one His creatures so filled with life, and so willing to pass it on to their child.

Once you feel a strong steady quality to this current of life zipping through the physical body of the child, hold your hands steady for a few moments to allow this pattern to become stably implanted. Become aware of your breathing. With each exhalation feel the intensity of the life-field increase. When you sense the pattern is complete, move on to the next physical contact point.

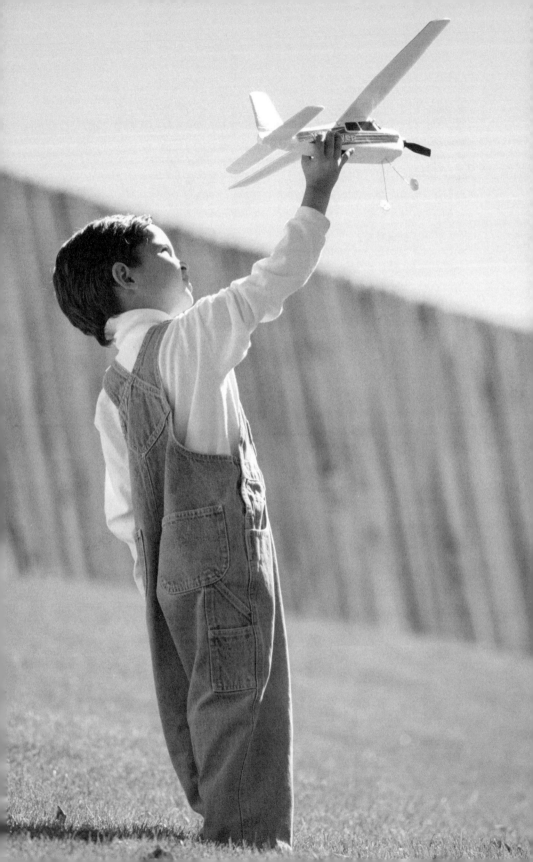

12

Radiance to the Thymus
The Spirit of Purity

The ability to purify ourselves is of vital importance in the age in which we live. Environmental toxins, sensory overstimulation, social violence and irresponsible governance create a poisonous context for our individual lives.

In our time, a heightened sense of the sacred is percolating to ever-wider circles of society, displacing the profane. We are in the midst of an Age of Purification in which the old ways are passing away. The old human order, created by the minds of humans divorced from cosmic wisdom, is plodding its last doddering steps towards the grave. The new spiritual order, which the babies of the future are responsible for stewarding, is coming into manifestation. At this point the human race as a whole has chosen life, rather than the extinction which would have been certain had we tethered our awareness to the old order and followed it into oblivion.

The interim period—before the full manifestation of the coming age—is a period of transition. The Earth is being purified. The mechanism by which this takes place is the purification of the Heaven. As the new Heaven takes form the Earth cannot help responding and following suit. Changes first happen in the Heaven, the invisible realm of consciousness, and are then reflected in the Earth.

Our focus, as awakened representatives of a new order, is less on changing the Earth than on changing the Heaven—the Heaven of our own consciousness. It is in the invisible realms that the purification takes place first. Once the purification has taken place in spirit, the world of form will follow effortlessly. If the spirit is right the form will follow.

The time of purification is the time in which many of the old forms will pass away. If we are attached to form it's painful. If our choice is to be with spirit we are agents of the Renaissance of spirit. There is a vast mass of material that requires transmuting in the fire of love. All the old creations of the human mind must go through the fires of purification to determine whether they can exist in the reborn world of love.

The thymus gland brings this spirit to particular focus in the physical body. After familiarizing yourself with the location of the thymus, celebrate the Spirit of Purity in your child.

§ § §

RADIANCE MEDITATION FIVE
THE SPIRIT OF PURITY: THE THYMUS

As you direct the life current from your hands into the area of the child's thymus, picture this area as a filter through which all the things in the old Earth must pass on their upward ascent. Only things which are right and pure and fitting can pass through the filter of purification to become part of the New Earth. The fire of love burning in the filter of purification incinerates all those things which have no place in the New Earth.

Anything at all that comes through your child's system must pass through the filter of purification. Anything polluting, anything poisonous, anything disruptive, anything that is less than the best that comes into your child's system will be incinerated by the Spirit of Purity. Picture your child remaining pure no matter what temptations, distortions, or negative influences might bombard it. See nothing being able to touch it which is not for the best.

Picture your child being able to walk through the very worst problems that you could ever imagine, and in shining purity emerge unscathed on the other side. Picture this child with a passion for purity which allows nothing unclean to enter in.

As you hold your hands steady over this point in the child's body, feel the Spirit of Purity take root and grow strong in the child. When you sense that this spirit is firmly rooted, move on to the next contact point.

§ § §

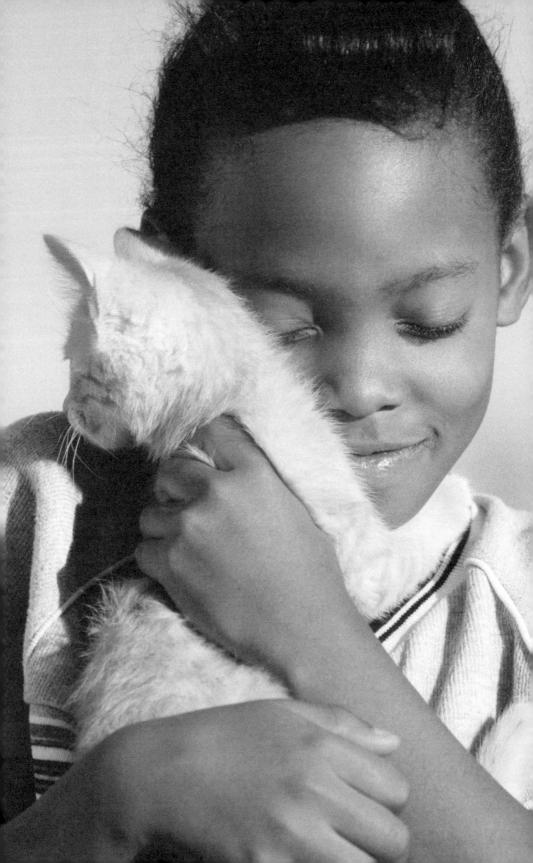

13

Radiance to the Islets
The Spirit of Blessing

If your child is a conduit for Radiant Love nurtured in the Womb of Truth, blossoming forth abundant Life and walking in perfect Purity, this child will bless the whole Earth. The spirit of blessing is a natural consequence of looking upon the face of God.

The blessed individual does not only receive blessing from God, the blessed individual is a blessing from God. The blessed person spreads blessing wherever they walk. Every hair on the head of the blessed one blesses the Earth. Every breath the blessed one breathes out, by mingling with the air on this planet, extends the radiance of God into the Earth. The one who is blessed cannot help but bless. The blessed one is so focused on giving blessing that there is no need to look for blessing. In the presence of a blessed one, blessing simply is.

Not only are the fellow human beings of a blessed one blessed, but God is blessed. Honor is given to God by the presence of a blessed one.

In the old Earth, blessing is seldom an inevitable product of human interaction. In the new Earth, blessing is the inevitable by-product of every interaction between human beings. Living in love, guided by truth, bursting with life, the women and men of Heaven cannot help but bless each other.

The Spirit of Blessing comes to a particular physical manifestation in the Islets of Langerhans. The Islets are a collection of endocrine cells dispersed throughout the pancreas. The pancreas is found adjacent to the ribcage, where the left elbow joint meets the torso (illustration in Chapter Eight).

§ § §

RADIANCE MEDITATION SIX
THE SPIRIT OF BLESSING: THE ISLETS OF LANGERHANS

Direct the energy flowing from your fingers towards a place on your child's body representing the Islets of Langerhans in the pancreas. As you do this, feel the Spirit of Blessing moving out from you with every outbreath. Allow the current of blessing to intensify and move more strongly through your hands each time you breathe out.

Fill your mind with the blessing this child will convey to every person they touch or even think of. Picture this child blessing the Earth and the natural world by their care and respect for spirit. Envision the pleasure God takes in the life of one who seeks to be a blessing to Him. Keep allowing this current of blessing to build each time you breathe out. Sense the current of blessing become strong and stable in the child. Hold this feeling for a few moments in quietness. Be blessed yourself by the blessing this child will be.

When you sense that the pattern of blessing is stable and strong in the child, move on to the next contact point.

§ § §

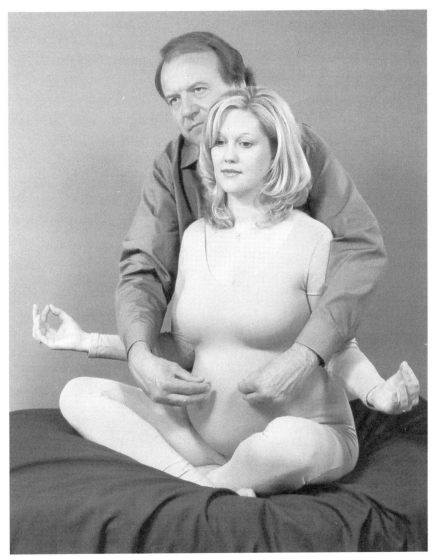

Radiance to the Islets

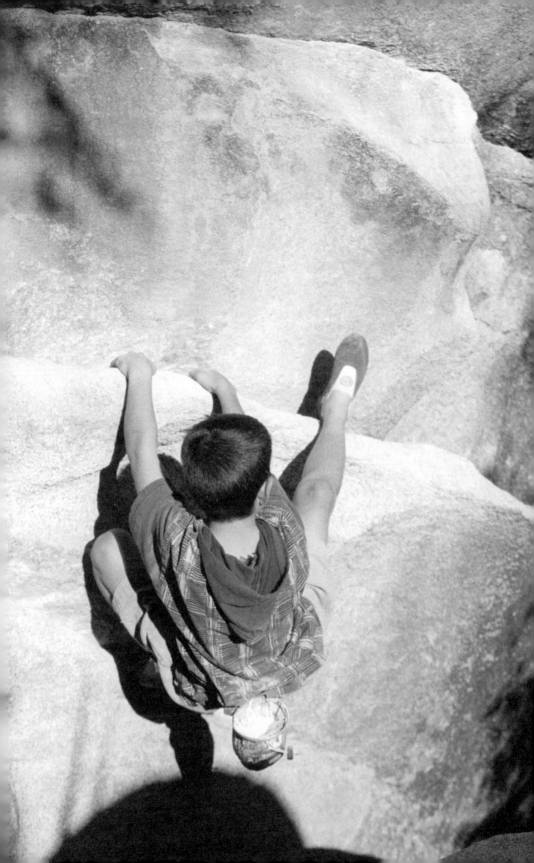

14

Radiance to the Adrenals
The Spirit of Purpose

The hormone secreted by the adrenal glands, adrenaline, brings the whole body into a heightened state of preparation for action. The spiritual essence of which this gland is the physical manifestation is the Spirit of Purpose. A child who embodies the Spirit of Purpose moves steadily toward his or her goal. Such a person is not distracted by his or her emotional compulsions, mental confusion, bodily wants, cravings or addictions.

The purposeful one is in control. The purposeful one is not pushed hither and yon by circumstance. The purposeful one is never "under the circumstances." The purposeful one acts in accordance with God's creative spirit springing up from within them, no matter what the outer circumstance looks like. No outside influences can disturb the Womb of Truth in which creation may take place in the world of the purposeful one. The eyes of the purposeful one are always fully directed at what they are looking at. Such a spiritual warrior is always fully in the moment, fully in control of his or her own incarnational vehicle. True control isn't about controlling people or events outside of yourself; it's about controlling the place from which your intentions and motivations spring, making sure that place is always your deepest inner integrity and wisdom.

The purpose served by the purposeful one is simple and constant: to worship God and to serve the whole of life. For the purposeful one, there are no agendas other than love and service. The purposeful one is charac-terized by singleness of purpose. In singleness of purpose, human wants and distractions are recognized and acknowledged, but are not placed in the position of control. The purposeful one never neglects messages com-ing from body, mind and heart, but also never lets those messages override the guidance of spirit.

What dictates behavior of the purposeful one is the creative pulsation of the moment, as it comes down from God out of Heaven. With eyes fixed singly on this goal, the purposeful one can bring the reality of Heaven into manifestation on Earth. The purpose of the purposeful one is never to attempt to please human beings. With singleness of mind the purposeful one directs her or his effort to pleasing God.

Only when there is double-mindedness and distraction is a person's vision fragmented, and fear enters in. Deceit and lies can never enter into the mind of one whose vision is singly centered in spirit. The vision of the one whose mind is purposefully fixed in spirit is radiant. It blesses all that it touches. When the fullness of divine purpose is known, the pettiness of human purpose becomes apparent and fades away.

Once your child becomes a blessing, the Spirit of Purpose directs that blessing into powerful manifestation in the outer world. In Radiance Meditation Seven, all the spiritual work done up to this point begins to move purposefully outward.

§ § §

RADIANCE MEDITATION SEVEN
THE SPIRIT OF PURPOSE: THE ADRENAL GLANDS

Become conscious once again of your breathing. Each time you breathe out feel the steadiness of your own life field. Feel the still point within you which is aligned with the Spirit of Love. When you feel your centering is as unwavering as the flame of a candle in a still room, move your hands down the child's body to a point which represents the adrenal glands. Use your spiritual sight to make accurate contact with this point.

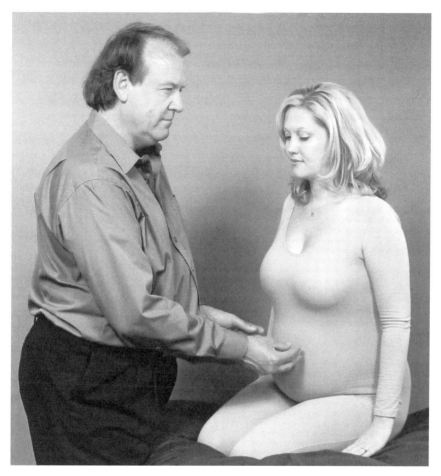

Radiance to the Adrenals

Using your breath as a guide, allow the current of the Spirit of Purpose to intensify in the radiation from your hands. Sense this spirit becoming fixed in the child. Welcome the Spirit of Purpose into the spiritual womb of the baby.

As you hold your hands above the adrenals in open welcome of the Spirit of Purpose, see the child moving in a straight line through life. Whatever the choices the child may have; whatever crossroads of experience the child may come to, see them choosing always the one which leads to the highest expression of divine purpose on Earth. See them meeting the fog of doubt, disappointment and dismay and moving through it with the steadiness of purpose known by one whose heart is centered in divine knowing.

Give thanks for the singleness of purpose of this child. Give thanks for the singleness of purpose with which its body is now growing in the womb. Know that it will bring this same singleness of purpose to its mental growth, its emotional growth, its growth of understanding of its own spiritual nature. May this child always know that its purpose is to shine the light upon the Earth.

When you sense a steadiness of radiance in this spirit, move to the next contact point.

§ § §

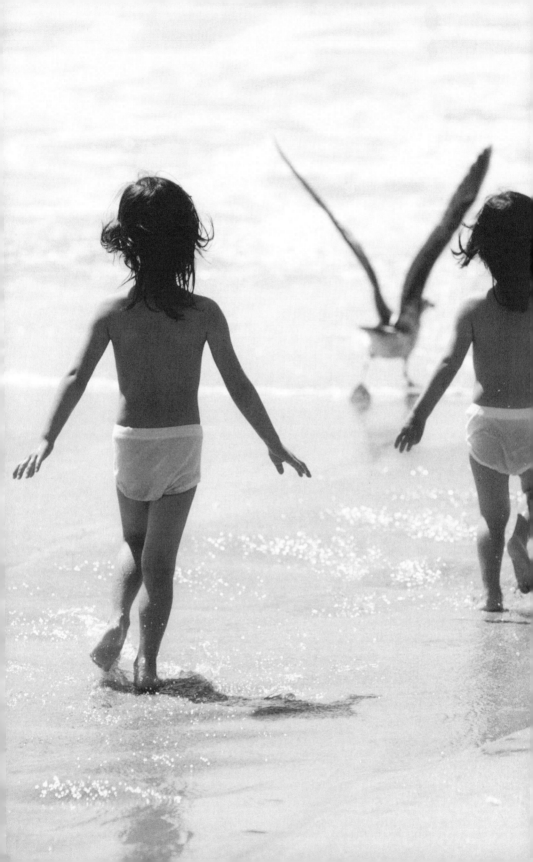

15

Radiance to the Gonads
The Spirit of Creation

The final endocrine glands, going from top to bottom, are the gonads, the sex glands. These are paired: in men, the testicles; in women, the ovaries. The Spirit associated with these endocrine glands is the Spirit of Creation.

Heaven is the realm of consciousness, out of which the Earth of form springs. When a new consciousness is present, humankind aligned with divine purpose, a new Heaven, the result is a new Earth. Trying to create a new Earth while keeping an old consciousness simply results in the same old cycle of conflict, betrayal and pollution. It is less the outside world that needs to be changed than the consciousness within you and me. When we fill ourselves with the new Heaven, the Spirit of Creation effortlessly brings forth the new Earth. Your growing child is a supreme work of the Spirit of Creation, bringing all the potential of the new Earth.

§§§

RADIANCE MEDITATION EIGHT
THE SPIRIT OF CREATION: THE GONADS

Move your hands to the next contact point. Keep this movement smooth and fluid, bearing in mind that your hands are touching the vibrational sphere of another being.

Sense when your hands have found the physical point that represents the gonads on the child's body. Envision the stream of bright love energy pouring from your hands into this point, and invoking the Spirit of Creation. With each outbreath, picture the flow of energy to this area becoming strong and stable. Welcome the Spirit of Creation into your own heart and mind.

As a minister of the new Heaven, this child will be an agent of divine beauty on Earth. This being will shed light by the very quality of its presence. Its actions will bring beauty. It will not be dominated by the old habits of mind and heart that enslaved past generations. It will no longer be bound by the boundaries that prohibited previous generations from being all that they could be.

This child will live without boundaries to its creativity. The presence of spirit welling up from within them will co-ordinate the unfoldment of everything around them. Each piece of their world will find its perfect place in the pattern of the whole of life.

As a child of the new Earth, this being will find itself listening for its cues not to peers, parents, habits, addictions, or the mass media, but to its inner voice. Its ear is always attuned to the messages that come from the Great Spirit. As it responds to these signals, it renews the Earth without trying, without striving. This child brings renewal simply by existing. With its heart rooted in the new Heaven, this child creates the new Earth.

Give thanks for the privilege of associating with this child, bringer of the new Earth. With each breath welcome the Spirit of Creation into the form of this child. Feel the Spirit of Creation becoming firmly implanted in the child's vibrational realm. When you sense that this flow is steady, gently move your hands on to the next contact point.

§ § §

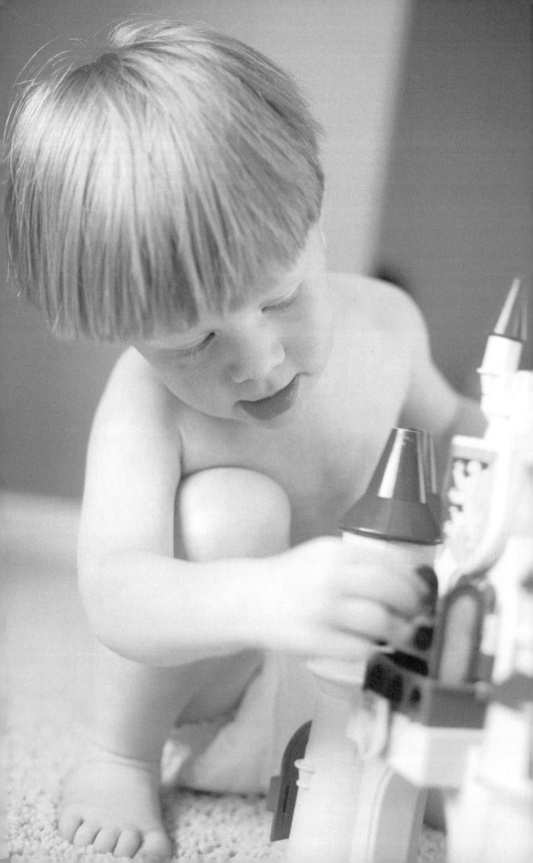

16

Radiance to Special Areas

O nce you have completed radiance to the gonads, the seventh and final set of endocrine glands, wrap up your time with this child by offering radiance to any area that requires special attention. The following Radiance Meditations guide you through these. After this, you conclude the session by going back to the Connection Point at the junction of the atlas and axis vertebrae.

There are several specialized areas which benefit from radiation, although they are not endocrine glands. Once we have established a steady flow of current through the endocrine glands, we can turn our attention to these other areas.

Hot Spots

During this phase of the radiation cycle, we can also use our sensitivity to spirit to locate any areas of the fetus' body that require special attention. This process is analogous to sensing, perhaps, that an adult has a bad back, or a faulty liver. We may "see" these conditions with our spiritual eyes. Our hands may pick up a pattern of turbulence, or disturbance of the energy flow. Such areas may feel "hotter," or icy "cold" as we move our hands over them. During the process of radiance we give these areas attention once the endocrine pattern is completed.

Infinite Connections

We can also offer radiation through one person to another. This whole process works unhindered at any distance. These Meditations can be done by the parents of a young child who is away from home. This is an excellent way to maintain a connection with an absent loved one. It is not dependent upon proximity in either time or space.

Radiance can also be offered to a fetus using the mother's body as the point of connection. In this case, attunement is given to both mother and child simultaneously. The same applies to the father.

Couples who share this kind of an attunement with each other regularly know that this is perhaps the most precious time they ever spend together. It communicates feelings and sensings too deep to be expressed. Our souls can speak at a level far beyond words. Even the words "I love you" presuppose an "I" and a "you"—a state of separation. Such distinctions disappear during a shared session of radiance.

In the current of radiance there is no separation, for no words are necessary. In this state we cannot fail to be aware of the underlying oneness of all things. The illusoriness of separateness is demonstrated by spirit, as it crosses freely between physical forms, hearts and minds in order to do its life-affirming work. Spirit knows no boundaries.

Radiance is also a useful practice for situations in which you are with people who are stressed. You don't have to say anything in order to have an impact on the situation. Radiance will offer a soothing influence to the inflamed mind and heart.

This applies equally well to your own mind and heart when they are disturbed. If you get yourself into a state of emotional distress, you aren't in a position to offer much healing or wisdom to those around you. Radiating to your own mind and heart will remind you of your spiritual origins. It centers you in the deepest core of your nature. It makes you aware that you have the resources of the universe at your disposal.

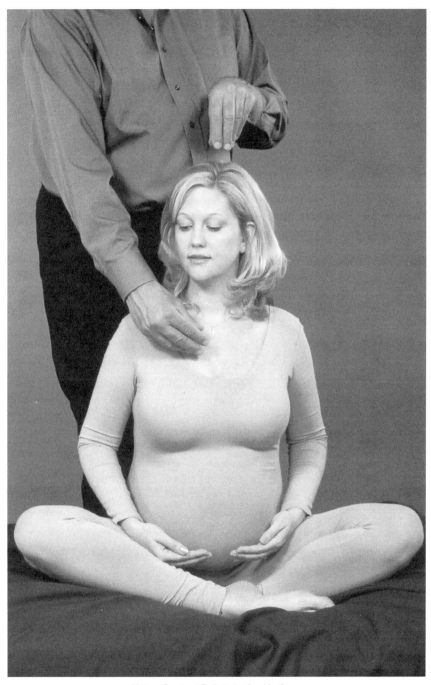

Using Contact Points in the Mother:
Radiance to the Thymus with Pineal as Contact Point

The ninth Radiance Meditation celebrates connection. We are all connected on the spiritual level to many other people. Through these heart links, we communicate constantly with others on an unconscious level. It is rather like a telephone switching station, with lines spreading out to many distant locations. What happens in the consciousness of the operator travels over all the lines simultaneously, to all the other people on our network.

When these kinds of messages come to us from people to whom we are connected, we may inexplicably feel depression, elation, fear, distress, or any number of other sensations and emotions. We pick up whatever they feel. If we are centered in right spirit, we simply send love back down the line. As creative beings, we choose not to reciprocate the distress! Radiance Meditation Nine deals with this special ability of living beings to interconnect with one another in a radiant spiritual network.

§ § §

RADIANCE MEDITATION NINE
THE SPIRIT OF THE WORLD: THE FRONTAL LOBES

Moving your hands carefully and respectfully through the child's vibrational substance, go to a point representing the upper front portion of the head, around the temples. Behind this area of the skull are the frontal lobes of the brain, the seat of much of our individuality and personality.

Open your hands once again (Hand Position B) as though you were cradling the front of someone's head. Allow your heart to fill with thanks for the individual nature of this precious child-to-be. Picture this one's individuality being expressed to the fullest and highest potential possible. Picture spirit breathing life into the individual nature of this child, nurturing it to become all it can possibly be.

Give thanks for the people that this child has already touched simply by existing. Give thanks for every contact it will have with other people throughout its life. Give thanks for the blessing this child will bring through everything it thinks, says, and does.

Treasure the preciousness of this child. Feel the substance of its world as it radiates from the frontal lobes out to your fingers and hands. Feel the intensity of the creative process going on within.

Allow the pressure of connection between you to build. As you cradle this sphere of spirit within your hands, picture strands of spirit going out to touch all the people this child will ever meet. Sense how these channels of connection with others will be conduits through which blessing may move out from this child. It will touch those who are connected with this strand whether or not their conscious mind is aware of it or whether the child is aware of it. Through our strands of connection with others we allow the spirits in our hearts to move out far beyond ourselves and affect hundreds of other individuals.

Feel your hands touching and blessing the child's entire world. Feel your hands touching and blessing the child's entire life. Feel the radiant current that comes from your hands touching and blessing every single person this child will every think about, talk about, be with or even glance at. When you have allowed the spirit of love to move through you fully to all these people, gently move your hands to the next contact point.

§ § §

Once you have focused on your child's relationship to the world, it is time to sense whether there are any particular organs that require spiritual attention. You may sense that a certain area needs more love or help. You may pick up a particular mental or emotional trait which could use a strengthening of the spiritual flow through it. You may feel that everything is working just fine. Whatever the case, it is appropriate to use your spiritual sensitivity to check out the child's vibrational patterns and to offer radiance wherever it is required.

§ § §

RADIANCE MEDITATION TEN
AREAS NEEDING SPECIAL ATTENTION

Moving very slowly, move your hands down the child's body. Feel how different areas of the body emit different vibrations. Sense which areas show great vibrational activity and which areas which are more dormant. Using your spiritual sight, and your hand's sensitivity to vibrations, "see" whether there are any areas of the child's body which seem to call out for your special love and care.

When you sense that there is a pattern of disturbance or turbulence, or perhaps just heightened intensity, around a certain organ or system, hold your hands over that place and maintain a steady current of radiation until you sense that the vibrational pattern is stabilized, or until you sense that you have done as much as you can in that area. This may be a few moments or half an hour. Use your innate sensing to tell you how long to dwell on each place. Don't get anxious and don't try to "fix" anything; simply share a cycle of love in each of these areas with the child.

If you sense that no particular area of the child's body is in turmoil, radiate up and down the whole physical form, giving thanks for its perfection. With each outbreath, let the baby feel your love and appreciation.

As you move your hands over the child's body, become acutely conscious of the silver thread that connects you upwards to Heaven and allow the creative energy pouring down this thread to bathe and encompass the child. As it is physically bathed in placental fluid, let its spiritual womb be bathed in the substance of love. The substance of love washes away all fear, and lets the processes of creation take place in all their flawless perfection.

§ § §

After attending to areas with special needs, the time comes to offer your blessing to the child's mind and heart.

§ § §

RADIANCE MEDITATION ELEVEN
MIND AND HEART

Picture the heart, the emotional realm of the baby. Picture this heart being still, and free of turmoil. Envision this child enjoying the gift of stillness of heart all its life long. May its stillness of heart be oil upon the troubled waters of human emotion; may it be able to see the unrippled reflection of the hearts of others in the still pond of its own quiet heart.

May its heart overflow with joy and giving and honesty. May the gift of its heart enrich the lives of those it meets. As the love of God pours down from Heaven to bathe this heart, may it overflow with love for others. May the love of God so fill this

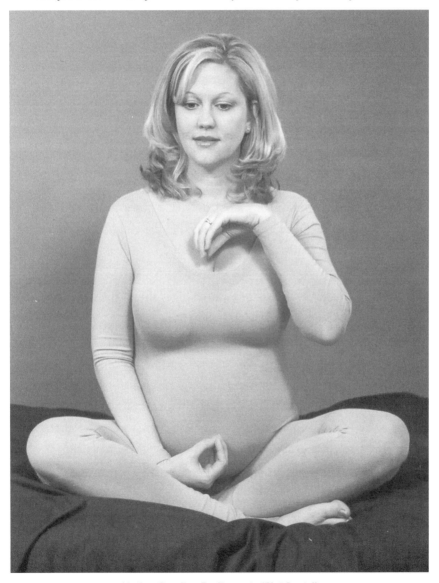

Mother Sending Radiance to "Hot Spots"

heart that there is no room for fear, anger, doubt, jealousy, resentment. May all negative emotions be washed away by the springing fountain of this heart's love.

Picture your child's love as a rich stream pouring forth in unending blessing. When this steam feels constant and secure, move your consideration to the child's mind. Allow an image of peace and stillness to fill your mind. Picture your child always having the gift of clarity of thinking, never being swayed by subconscious compulsions, emotional outbursts, or unthinking habits.

Let this child's mind dwell only on the light. As it dwells on the light, it becomes the bearer of the light; the bringer of divine light into the affairs of men. May the clarity of its perception guide this child through all the deceptions and pitfalls of the old world. May its wisdom illuminate the new Heaven and the new Earth.

§ § §

When you sense through your hands that the pattern of clarity of mind and stillness of heart is firm and stable in the child, move your hands to the final contact point.

We end each session of radiance where we began: the area of the atlas and axis vertebrae, the Crossover Point. This is always the way a session is concluded. The circle returns to its origin point.

You will usually experience a marked difference from your first visit to the Crossover Point, at which you began this time of radiance. The intensity of spirit moving through the baby will often feel much clearer and more powerful, like a swift, unobstructed stream. Your own energy has almost always increased a great deal, and your sensitivity is heightened. It is important to close every session in this way.

§ § §

RADIANCE MEDITATION TWELVE
THE CROSSOVER POINT REVISITED

Move your hands gently back to the point where you first began to offer radiation at the base of the skull. Hold your hands in such a

*way that they focus the beam of your vibration-energy (Hand
Position A). This point represents the junction between the New
Heaven and the New Earth. This is the point through which the
qualities of Heaven flow through into the Earth. This is the point
through which all the spirits move from potential into manifestation.
Picture this channel being clear of any obstruction, and wide enough
to let the fullness of this child's spirit move down into its form.*

*Hold this vision for a few moments until this channel is work-
ing swiftly and efficiently. When you feel that this is so, become
aware of your breathing. Feel, with each outbreath, spirit flowing
into form. As you inhale, absorb all the intensity of God's love flowing down out of Heaven through the connection through the top of
your head.*

*Spend a few moments allowing this energy to move where it
needs to move. Absorb the sparkling rain of energy into every par-
ticle of your being. Feel it refreshing you and re-invigorating every
cell in your body. Give thanks for the strength and potency of this
divine connection. Give thanks for being one of those who has the
privilege of consciously knowing their divine connection.*

*Ask in your heart if there is anything else that Spirit would
have you know. Know that you can dwell in this state of being, this
state of grace and bliss, throughout the day, simply by becoming
aware of the existence of it. Feel your body breathing in and out, in
and out, in and out. When you are ready, open your eyes.*

§ § §

Attuning to the Implicate Order of Life

Spiritual contact with the unborn child ought to be an ongoing
process. Parents should check in with the fetus at least once a day or more,
just to make sure that all the vibrational patterns are developing smooth-
ly. With experience, this process becomes almost instinctive.

This time of the day becomes a deeply sacred period of connection
and affirmation of the child's spirit. It becomes something that one would
neglect no more readily than feeding a child, or washing it. Once the

importance of spiritual factors is recognized, these in fact become more important than the outer circumstances.

With practice, our eyes become sharp, our ears become tuned, to the spiritual nature of things. We no longer look for causes on the physical level. We seek the origins of things—emotions, events, diseases—on the invisible level at which they originate. The creative process always begins on the invisible level, and moves to the visible. After a time, we are no longer distracted by the visible, and do our most significant work in the realm of spirit.

The ability to pick up the invisible factors present in any situation becomes not second nature, but first nature. Our concern with manipulating the material world in order to secure our satisfaction fades into the past as we recognize that spirit already has the world under control: there is a pattern inherent in life itself. As we identify our outer selves—our incarnational vehicles of body, mind and heart—with life, that inherent order flows out through our actions.

Only trust is required, trust that life works. And that should be the first thing that having a baby teaches us: Life works!

PART FOUR

The Child Restored

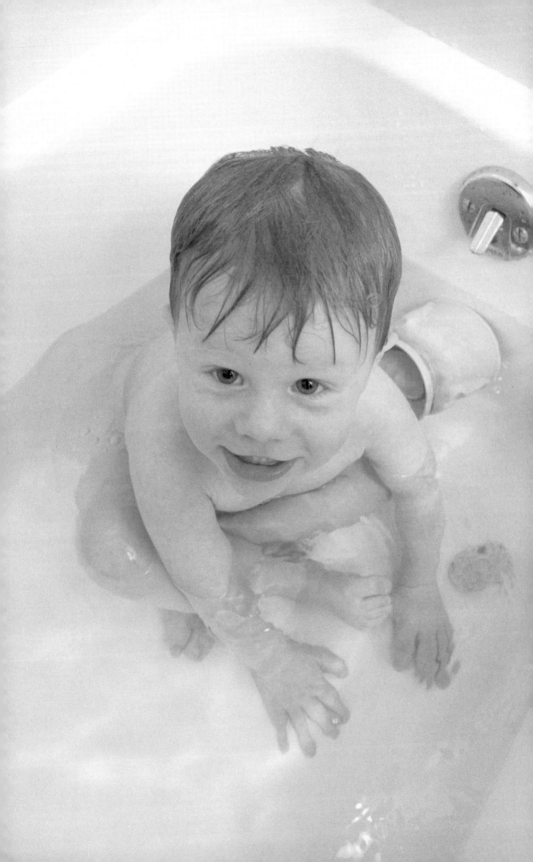

17

Spiritual Roles of Father and Mother

Every common action has a mythic dimension. When we as individuals repeat certain actions that millions of other individuals have done over time, we participate in the archetype of that particular action. The ancient Greeks represented archetypes in their literature in such a vivid way that they are still with us today: Hydra, Oedipus, Aphrodite, and many others.

The Mother As Archetype

Parenting is a mythic event. A woman is not merely a solitary mother of a single child. Through childbirth, through simply being a woman, she participates in the myth of the Great Mother. The qualities of the Great Mother are known: infinite caring, inexhaustible tenderness, fierce protection of her young, bringing forth Earth's bounty, and replenishing the species. A woman participates in these age-old realities simply by being herself.

The characteristics of these myths are passed from generation to generation. They are passed from mother to child. If they are weakly represented in the mother, they may be weakly represented in the child. If the mother is a strong example of the qualities of the Great Mother, there will be a strong image in the child's mind of what this means. Once implanted in the child's reasoning, these values come out in all the child's dealings with, and vision of, the world.

Part of the feminine model is the essence of caring. This great archetype of a caring mother transfers readily from the child's early experience into the child's later relationships with other people, and with all living things. For example, a child with a strong assumption of the values of the Great Mother will be able to relate to our planet as the Earth Mother. Such a person could never harbor the idea that personal survival depends on exploiting the planet. The mental circuitry for this sort of assumption is simply not there. Destroying the environment for personal gain will not be an option for such a child.

In this way we program into our children the assumptions we program into ourselves. If we remain unhealed ourselves, we cannot offer our children healing. Conversely, as we let ourselves be healed first, we are able to extend healing to our children. The actions of a healed one spread out with a ripple effect, and ultimately extend healing to the entire planet.

A healed child, with a vivid subconscious picture of the qualities of the Great Mother, will give all women the respect due the Great Mother. Such a child will see the Great Mother reflected in all women, and will honor them accordingly.

Earth Mother Represents Heaven Mother

To her children, the earthly mother is a representation of the Great Mother in living flesh. She is the Goddess made manifest. She is a flesh representation of the essence of Woman. She is a living monument, a walking icon of Godhead in its female form. If she faithfully represents this in all her actions, the child will be able to relate to all the other places in human relations where this archetype is found. If there is a void where this Goddess-image should be, there will be a void in relating to others in this way. A nurturing childhood anchors the child against the force of all the distortions that arise from the outside world and the mass subconscious.

So true motherhood is not an everyday commonplace happening. It is an event of mythic proportions! In motherhood, woman becomes the living flesh representation to the child of Mother God. Without this example, there will a void in the child's conceptual world where the image of Mother God should be.

Heavenly Father in Earthly Form

To his children, the earthly father is a representation of their Heavenly Father. A child is not adept at separating spirit from flesh. A child lives in the awareness of the union of the two: Heaven gives rise to Earth, and Earth ascends to Heaven; Heaven and Earth are one. A child is not capable of reasoning: "Ah, now, my earthly father is doing these awful things, but my Heavenly Father would never do that." To the child, seeing Heaven and Earth interchangeably, there is no bold line dividing earthly and Heavenly Father. The earthly father is the concrete flesh representation to the child of the Heavenly Father. The spiritual responsibility of the earthly father is to represent the qualities of the Heavenly Father accurately to the child.

The earthly father cannot create this model of Father God out of his own wisdom and strength. The only way in which an earthly father can represent Father God to his children is by becoming one with his Heavenly Father. The earthly father allows his personal ego to fade, his personal identity to diminish, to the point where he is transparent. When his earthly personality fades into insignificance as his full attention is turned to his Heavenly Father, he becomes one with his Heavenly Father. His earthly life becomes a transparency through which his Heavenly Father is clearly seen. The earthly father who has blended his identity in joyous union with his creator is a window through which the light of Heaven may shine.

The Focus of the Hero

How does the earthly father do this? By love. His paramount love is for his Heavenly Father. He shows his love for his Heavenly Father by doing His works, by the care he takes to be a faithful steward of his Heavenly Father's creation. Consumed in love for his Heavenly Father, his earthly personality fades into the distance. When others look at him, they see only the face of the Father within.

The source of inspiration and causality for the earthly father is not his wife, his children, or anyone around him. The face of his attention is instead turned always to the Heavenly Father within. When and only when the earthly father's response is first and foremost to the Great Father, the love of the Great Father shines out from him to bless those around him.

To his children, the earthly father is the flesh representation of the Heavenly Father. As his children grow into understanding, they easily recognize the qualities of Heaven wherever in life they find them, for they have known from birth the representation of Heaven.

Boy children with such a father know what manhood is about, for they have seen the example of a man consumed with love for the things of Heaven. They have lived with a father though whose eyes they could look and see God. They know what true manhood means. They are not likely to be sidetracked by violent, uncaring, or macho stereotypes of "manhood" they may encounter in the mass culture.

Girl babies, as they grow up, also know what true manhood is about. They can sense it, or the lack of it, in the men they meet. For they have seen the form of their Heavenly Father shining through the presence of their earthly father. They are unlikely to be mislead by "men" who posture impressively; who talk grandly, who look good on the outside but are empty husks at the core. They are accustomed to seeing through a man.

The earthly father welcomes anyone to see through him, for in doing so they can gaze upon the face of the Great Father within. Being "seen through" is no threat for the man whose response is anchored in the Father within.

The True Responsibility of Parents

With an earthly mother representing the Womb of Truth, and an earthly father representing the face of Love, the child of Life can be born. The child of spirit-filled parents has a complete spiritual education through witnessing the Being of its parents.

Once Being is in place, all other earthly skills required can be added. If Being is not in place, is not understood, then no matter how many earthly skills a child may acquire, the central core of that child will never be firm. Our present society teaches us to acquire goods and expertise. This is an unsatisfying attempt to substitute forms for the central reality of spirit.

The primary responsibility of the parent is not to give the child a good school, a nice house, and material stimulation. The primary task of the responsible parent is to represent spirit to the child. Children soon see if their parents' emphasis is on the inner reality or outer forms, and begin to structure their own reality accordingly.

Wealth does not bring security. Material goods do not bring security. What does bring security is knowing who you are, and knowing that what you are on the deepest level is God. Once the reality of God-Being is experienced, and the conviction of oneness with a friendly universe is absolutely fixed in place, then the child may remain a poor peasant, or sit in the councils of the mighty, and neither external condition affect his or her sense of self.

The only thing that matters to the child of God is that they live in God. There is no other reality. There is no other fulfillment. Parents who live in God represent the reality of God living in the flesh to their children. This is spiritual parenting.

Replacing Absent Archetypes

There are few people who have healthy archetypes of the Great Mother and Great Father instilled during their childhood experiences. How do we then develop and heal these aspects of ourselves, so that we can pass them along to our children?

Rewiring our consciousness is no small matter. For each of us to have a functioning archetype of the Great Mother and Great Father, we have to undo much of what we learned at an early age.

The following meditation is designed to start the ball rolling, initiating the process of healing. It is a profound experience, and one that may trigger much reflection and many life-changes.

For this Exercise, make sure you are in a quiet room and will not be disturbed. Low lights are helpful, as is quiet, meditative music. You can tape the Eighth Exercise and play it back to yourself, or use the downloadable audio version. Alternately, have your partner or a friend read it to you.

§ § §

EIGHTH EXERCISE
REVISIONING MOTHER & FATHER GOD

Close your eyes. Let your whole body become still. Breathe deeply, and feel the tensions drain out of your body. Become aware of each inbreath and each outbreath. Visualize the tension in your body as a colored fluid, filling every part of you. As you breathe out, let more of this colored fluid out with every breath.

Start at your feet. With each outbreath, visualize the tension leaving your feet, breath by breath. Keep breathing out the colored tension-fluid until your feet are completely relaxed. Feel how empty and loose your feet are. Enjoy the feeling of emptiness.

When you have drained every molecule of tension out of your feet, and they are completely relaxed, start on your calves. Let the fluid filling your calves and ankles move out of you on your breath,

breath by breath, until they are completely empty and relaxed. When every cell in your calves is relaxed, move on to your thighs.

Do this all the way up your body. Drain your shoulders of the colored tension-energy, letting them sag completely. Once you have breathed out all the fluid and they are completely relaxed, start with the top of your head and begin to breathe out all the tension in your head. Let all the struggles of this day recede. Let all the thoughts and concerns of this day glide gently out of your body as you breathe out. Take as many breaths as you need to let all the tension energy out of your head.

Then clear your mouth and neck, allowing the last bits of tension to flow out of you. Now, with your whole body limp and relaxed, let your attention drift down again to see if you have any pockets of colored tension-energy that linger still. Find those subtle areas where you are still tense, and allow these last lingering tensions to slip gently out of your body with each relaxed breath.

You are now an empty, relaxed physical form. Behind you, sense the beautiful radiant presence you are coming to know quite well. It is the real you, the angel that is the truth of your being. Take a moment to appreciate the beauty of your spiritual self. Feel your body being enfolded in the radiant presence of this loving spirit. Feel the wonderful sense of fulfillment and completion that comes when the inner you and the outer you become one.

Notice how your spirit-body is connected upward, a bright cord that comes out of the top of your head and reaches all the way up to Heaven. Through this cord, feel the love of Heaven flowing down to you. Feel your own thankfulness at being one with this wonderful being flowing upwards up the cord.

Once you have had ample time to enjoy the miracle of oneness, call up before you a series of images, like a movie of your life, scene by scene. Linger on those memories that are most vivid. Re-experience them fully. Feel what it felt like to be there. Remember all the feelings associated with each scene. Keep going back, further and further, till you are a youth, a child, a baby. Go back to the earliest memories of childhood.

Think of an incident when you were a child, a time when you had a really great experience of meeting a wonderful man. Think of the man that impressed you most when you were very young. Just remember how awed you were to be meeting such a man. Remember the feeling of importance that you had, just being in the presence of this man. Remember the feeling. Pause for a moment to re-create that feeling fully. Hold that feeling with you strongly.

Now imagine the light of connection shining down from Heaven on to this man's head, the light of connection to Father God. Visualize this man really loving you as a child, and treating you as though you were the most important person he had ever met. See his love for you. Visualize Father God's love pouring out to you through the eyes of this man. When you have a very strong picture of being loved and respected and treasured and honored in this way, let the image fade, but let the feeling of being loved and soothed by this wonderful man remain.

Now think back to another thing that happened when you were a child. Think back to the worst experience you had with an adult man. Think of the meanest, cruelest man, perhaps someone who abused you terribly, or perhaps someone who you just saw but knew was bad. Remember how frightened you felt. Remember how power-less you were against this awful man. Remember how small you were. Remember all the worst things that happened. Remember all the feelings that went along with those awful things you experienced.

Now picture the wonderful man coming down from above, into the place where you are with the horrible man. As he comes down, light comes from his body. He is looking at you with love. You feel his love. You feel all the wonderful things you felt before in his presence. You feel safe, secure, protected by his shining presence. You run to him and he embraces you and enfolds you safely in his shining presence.

You look back again at the horrible man, but he is fading away! As the light streams into the place from the beautiful man, the awful man is like a shadow that is just melting away. You can hardly see him anymore. There is nothing to be afraid of anymore! You feel how much stronger the power of the wonderful man is than that of the horrible man. You take the hand of the Great Father and walk towards where the awful man was. But there is nothing there anymore. He is like a dark shadow that faded away when the light of your True Father appeared. You look into the eyes of your father, and they are full of love for you. You know that he will always be there when you need him. You know he can always protect you. You know he can always dispel the forces of darkness.

Now go back to the movie of scenes from your life. Find a picture, a particular image, that represents your earthly father. It could be a photograph, or a particular memory, or even a feeling that you had when you were around him. Just choose something that sums up your father for you.

Now picture his face really closely. Picture looking into his eyes. Feel the feelings you felt when you were around him.

Now let his face and his eyes dissolve into the face and eyes of the Great Father. Even as you are watching, the contour of his face changes and blends into the face of the Great Father. Feel the love your father had for you. Maybe he wasn't able to show it, maybe he never expressed it, but know that he was trying to love you the best he knew how. He may not have known the best way. But he was trying. Feel how much he wanted you to know how he loved you, even if he never showed it.

Feel yourself loving him back. Feel how full your heart is with the Great Father's love. Feel how loving you feel towards your earthly father, and how much you appreciate his having tried so hard. Feel your love just pouring over him. Feel how much the Great Father loves him. Feel the Great Father's love melting your daddy's heart. See his heart being caught up into the heart of the Great Father. Just watch, and give thanks, for as long as you like. Enjoy seeing your daddy and the Great Father become one.

Now go back to your movie of your life as a child. If there are any scenes you would like to go where there were bad experiences with men, feel the terror of them fully. Then allow your Great Father to be there with you, and feel the peace and serenity that comes from his presence. Know he will always be there for you. Turn the tape off till you are done with remaking your childhood men. You can turn it on again when you are ready to go on.

§ § §

When you have remade as many scenes from your childhood as you like, think back to the most wonderful experience with a woman that you had. Remember a time when you were very young, and were with a woman who you thought was just wonderful. Remember how awed you were at her presence. Remember how beautiful and graceful she seemed. Remember how good she was to other people. Remember how good that child that is you felt just to be with her. Keep feeling that feeling. Treasure that feeling in your heart, and keep it in your memory.

Now envision that stream of light from Heaven shining down on the top of her head, making her whole body glow with light. She becomes more and more beautiful as the light pours down upon her. Her face, her eyes, her hair, her body all shine with beauty.

Now picture her eyes turning to look at you, the child. They are the eyes of Mother God. You feel the Truth of who she is, you feel the absolute trust you have for her spirit. You feel how enfolded you are in her presence. Engrave this feeling on your heart.

When you have the feeling firmly fixed in your heart, let the image fade, and see your movie of your life once again. As you review the scenes, pick a time when you had a horrible experience with a woman as a young child. Picture the scene and remember how it was. Remember exactly what happened. Recall every detail of the scene, and just how bad it was. Remember how awful you felt inside.

Now see the Great Mother coming down from Heaven. As she comes down, the whole place where you are is filled with radiant light. Her presence brings a lightness, a joy, a perfection with it. You look at her and feel the awful feeling in your heart melting. She reaches her hand down to take yours, looking at you with love. You feel your heart jump up to be with her, to join with her.

You look back now to where the horrible woman was, but she is dissolving in the light coming from Mother God. Your fear has melted, and you walk towards her, but there is nothing but a shadow left. You walk right through the spot where she was. There is nothing there anymore.

You look up into the eyes of Mother God, and know that she will always be there for you, whenever you need her. You know that her Truth will dispel any falsehood, and you can call on the Great Mother to represent Truth to you whenever you are in doubt. Know that you will always be able to remember this feeling whenever you need it.

Now go back to your movie. Find an image that represents your earthly mother: a photograph, a scene, perhaps even an object. Find whatever it is that really represents your mother to you. Now feel the feelings that you associate with this image of your mother.

Feel them fully. Feel the way you felt about her when you were a child. Remember the way she was towards you.

When you have this image of your earthly mother firmly in your mind, imagine a light coming from behind the image. It makes the whole image light. The image glows with radiance. Through the image of your mother shines the light of the Great Mother. Feel again how much the Great Mother loves you. Feel her love pouring to you through the image of your mother. Feel the spirit that you know is true of Mother God. Envision Mother God and your earthly mother blending into one.

Spend some time, now, to be with your earthly mother. See how hard she was really trying, despite the burdens that she had to deal with. See how the light was really shining inside her, although it was buried so much of the time. Let the light in you connect with the light in her, and let your two lights mutually reinforce each other.

When you have enjoyed some time with the true spirit of your mother, go back to the movie of your childhood. Remember any other miserable or frightening times you had with adult women. Be fully in them. Remember all the feelings they brought up in you. Then invoke the light of Mother God. Let Her be there in the situation with you. Feel again the feelings you have in Her presence.

When you have dealt with as many situations as you like, become aware of your radiant beam of connection upward with the light. Feel the light streaming down on you from Heaven. Let the essences of Mother God and Father God pour down into you with the light. Let the essence of Mother God take root in your heart. Find a special place in your heart where the essence of Mother God belongs, and put it there. Let this be the holy place you can always go back to when you need to remember the Great Mother.

Let the essence of Father God fill you as the light streams down from above. Let the essence of Father God take root in your heart. Find a part of your heart that belongs exclusively to Father God. Let the essence of Father God rest there, to blossom into your awareness whenever you need Him. Remember this most sacred place where God the Father will always live in you.

Keeping the intensity of this feeling with you, spend a few moments radiating the spirit of Father God and Mother God to people who you know who particularly need it. Think of friends and relatives who are not in touch with the spirit of either Father God or

Mother God, or both, and visualize a current of your radiance reaching out to them, wherever they are on the surface of the planet. The distance doesn't matter. See the radiance touching their hearts, breathing into their experience the essences of Mother and Father God. Bless them with your radiance. Feel them bathed in your love.

When you are done, let the pattern of radiance come to rest. Feel your spirit become still again. Let the glow around you become regular and steady. Become aware of your breathing. Feel your breath traveling in and out. When you are ready, open your eyes. Let the way you feel at this moment stay with you the whole day. Look for ways to radiate the essence of Father God or Mother God to the people you meet. Go back to those two special places in your heart whenever you need to.

§ § §

Unlimited Grace For Unlimited Healing

We can re-create the perfect father and the perfect mother within our own psyche, within our own lifetime, by exposing ourselves to the kind of healing work found in the above Exercise.

We do not have to be bound by the imperfect stereotypes that we have constructed out of personal experience and the mass consciousness. Some of us as children had inadequate experience, miserable experience or no experience of what true earthly parents should be. There is a void in our psyche where these life-creating symbols should be. If this void remains, life will continue in us unfulfilled.

But this does not mean that we cannot restore these cornerstones to our lives. We don't have to live all our lives without the Great Mother and Father God, and the destructive effect this has on our personal relationships. The psychological scars inflicted upon us as children do not have to remain in our consciousness, where they are likely to be re-inflicted on our own children. We can be healed.

Father and Mother God exist in spirit even though they may not exist in form in our awareness. As we begin to live in spirit ourselves, we suddenly have access to all the things we lack in form. And as the spirit grows strong in our experience and becomes habit, becomes first nature, spirit begins to fill out the forms that our necessary. The desolate places of our experience are comforted. The weak places are made strong. Mourning becomes joy. Grief and lack are replaced by fulfillment and peace. We are rebuilt, reconstructed in Life's perfect image as we come close to Love and Truth.

We can be completely restored. That doesn't mean just being patched up enough to continue functioning. It means claiming the glorious fullness of life. The old scars in mind and heart can melt. Our innermost being can be transformed. As we live with Father and Mother God in spirit, their presence reaches down into form to transform our lives, our work, our relationships. If you didn't have this example represented to you by adults when you were a child, spirit can put it there. Spirit can overcome all things.

Once we are healed, and we learn to live our lives and go our way as spiritually responsible and mature adults, we look for opportunities to radiate spirit to others. As this becomes a natural and normal thing to do, a common habit, it has a powerful effect on the body of mankind.

Being God to the Child

Myths are the shared race memory of the species. As we live our lives as heroes and heroines, being God in our circumstances, the energy field created by our actions reinforces the whole energy field of similar actions on the planet. In this way, we co-create the new myths, the myths of humankind restored to its true position of oneness with God. As enough individuals change their own reality, the reality of the whole is changed, and the Earth is returned once again to its creator.

As we as individuals take responsibility for being reborn ourselves, we offer the gift of immaculate conception to our children. They are no longer born just out of human heritage. As we allow ourselves to blend with God, we allow them to be born of spirit and flesh simultaneously, fruit of the union of God and humans.

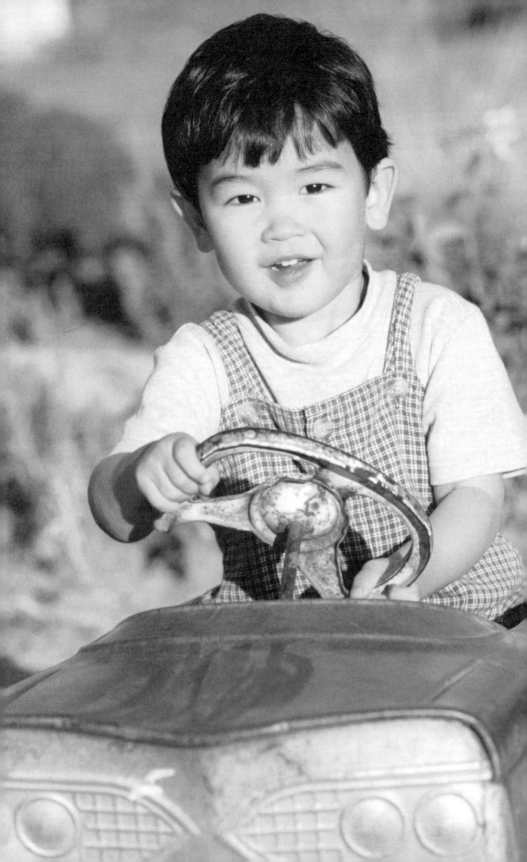

18

Spirit-Filled Relationship

As the previous chapter shows, healing of the child begins with healing of the parent. In order for the parent to extend wholeness to the child, the parent must be whole to start with. You can offer only what you have. The advent of a child is the catalyst for spiritual renewal in ourselves. As we consider birth, we must consider first of all our own rebirth.

The Power of Transcendent Relationship

A child is God's calling card. Coming into the world full of potential, full of newness, a child is a living reminder of our own need for newness, an invitation to reconsider our own potential.

The fact that, in a spiritual relationship, the substance of both parents is required to create the climate for the birth of spirit into the world through a child, forces us as parents to re-examine our relationship with each other.

What is the quality of our being together? Do we put spirit first, or are we centered in the world of form? Do we spend our time objecting to the outer form of our partner's behavior, or do we discern the inner essences? A fetus growing in the inmost part of the body is a powerful symbol of the creativity that hides in the inner parts of us. Honoring the spirit of the unborn child is an expression of our desire to honor the most sacred parts of our own inner nature.

Relationships between men and women are one of the primary areas in which the most vivid contrasts of human behavior are found. They inspire people to the most noble as well as the most depraved behaviors. People can assume a pleasant veneer which suffices for casual social relationships, but those they live with day in and day out see the flaws that are hidden from general view. In this way partnering and parenting relationships go to the core of what we really are, to the roots of being.

If we are able to have victory in the dark corners of our lives, the light that is released illuminates every other area more brightly. If the quality of our integrity stands up to the gaze of even those who have most frequent opportunity to witness our failures, we stand tall indeed. It is in these relationships that our subtle weaknesses are exposed. They are consequently our most valuable proving ground for practical spirituality.

When your relationship with your partner is a transcendent one, it is a source of deep power and affirmation on both the inner and outer level. Couples that have learned the lessons of living together with joy possess a magical resource infinitely more important than any outer possession.

These relationships are where the real spiritual work is done of restoring the Earth to Life. They are the first place we demonstrate our degree of personal awakening. It is not the teachers, orators, swamis, and preachers who do the great work of enlightenment. It is the people in the trenches: those who show the face of God to the world by their everyday actions. It is people who stand in the checkout line at the supermarket with grace, who lubricate axle bearings with serenity, who clean up after bedridden patients with a spirit of love, who mow lawns with the voice of God singing in their minds.

The Veneer of Pleasantness

The quality of our most private relationships is not a hidden thing. It may not be visible to many people. But it shows up at the forefront of our spirit. Anyone can appear pleasant to a stranger. But how do you appear to your partner, first thing in the morning? Do you radiate love, acceptance, joy and peace? Are you an inspiration to the world with the first words you say? Are the first thoughts that you allow into your mind ones which bring Heaven into the Earth?

Parenting brings all these issues to point. To create a spiritual womb for the child, our own spirits must be clear. Clear creation is done through a clear spirit. A spirit contaminated with judgment, blame, criticism and accusation will contaminate the creations which spring in to form through it. Spirit underlies form. Form reflects spirit—faithfully. That is why trying to clean up displeasing forms is futile. If we pay attention to the quality of spirit that we put out, taking care that it is clear, then our creations in form will be clear. The radiance of spirit will shine through them.

What parent would not want the light of Heaven to shine through their child? The parent that wants this has a direct personal responsibility. The light of Heaven shines through the child when it is allowed to shine through the pure heart and still mind of the parent. And that means saying "No!" to all the dark things that rise up from within us to obscure our light, and cast a shadow upon our children.

These dark things are most often jarred loose by our most intimate personal relationships. Husbands and wives typically talk to each other in tones much less sensitive than those they employ with anyone else they know. They reserve their harshest criticism for each other. They feel a license to abuse each other that they are not granted in other relationships. They are short with each other, dismissive, and oblivious to change. They are often the first to resist and the last to notice growth in the other.

It is extremely paradoxical that in relationship with the ones we claim to love most, the veneer of civility is thinnest. We talk to them more rudely than to anyone else we know. And supposedly we love them the most! If closeness were judged by the way we talk to each other, an objective observer might conclude that our husbands and wives are the people we love least!

This is why these relationships are the most fertile field for spiritual renewal. It is no accident that these relationships are the closest to us. It is no accident that these are the people we are with most of the time. The reason for this close association is that this is where the real, deep spiritual work is done. Life has designed things in such a way that we are presented with our most radical opportunities for growth in our most obvious relationships. We don't have to climb the Himalayas to Lhasa. We don't have to crawl the Stations of the Cross. Our sanctity is shown instead by the way we treat those who are closest to us everyday.

Our most sacred relationships are not those we have with our gurus, shamans, priests or pastors. Our most sacred relationships are those we have with our partners. They are designed to give us the most practice in being holy. They give us constant opportunities to transcend our petty emotions. They are full of room for the expression of the light-beings of spirit that we are. When we are expressing our light constantly in these relationships, we are truly filled with light.

How is this accomplished?

Choosing Love

Our choices are made in the moment. They are not made to cover the future. The future is the sum of all the instants that we create. It is by being light in these present moments that we shed light into the future.

In the moment that a situation comes up in which we are habitually inclined to show our fangs, we choose to show our halo instead. Each time we would instinctively lash out at our loved one, we choose instead to love.

The love is inside us, after all. The love is in fact the truest part of us. Bitterness and anger may dwell in our hearts too. But expressing it only reinforces that habit pattern. Every time we choose to love rather than choosing to fear, we strengthen the habit of love. The sum total of our choices determines our character.

Negative habit patterns may be very deeply ingrained. Fortunately, we do not have to deal with the whole pattern at once. We only have to deal with the present moment. Each time that habit comes up, we have an opportunity to make our choice in that moment. We either say: "Yes, I will bow down and worship at the shrine of this habit by giving in to it" or we say, "I recognize this habit, and know it exists in a part of me. But I also know that in essence I am an angel. I choose to express the angel."

We choose what we express. And in time, we become what we express. The things we allow to come through us, mold us. As we begin to consistently choose the angel in each moment, that choice becomes a habit. We turn first to Heaven in any situation, because we have forgotten how to engage the negative emotions that once were our staple. The sum total of an infinite number of present moments becomes our weeks, our years, our lifetimes.

In choosing Heaven as the source of our actions, we begin to bring Heaven into the Earth. We become identified with Heaven. As we drop the behaviors that are our human grave clothes, we become one with the nature of Heaven. "Heaven" no longer means an ephemeral afterlife. It is the stuff of everyday reality. Every day is filled with opportunities to express the character of Heaven. In this way, the Earth is reclaimed for its Creator.

PART FIVE

The Lessons of Fifteen Years

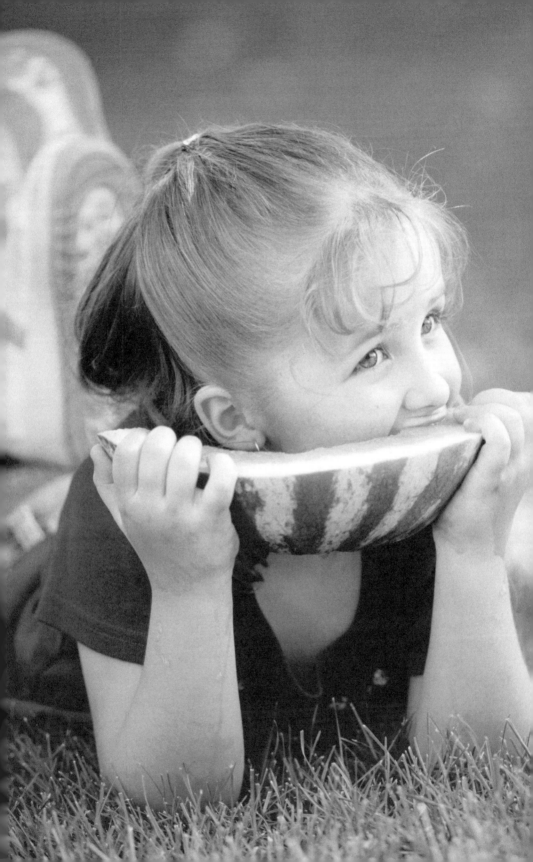

19

My Journey In Parenting

Parenting without a spiritual base can be a wrenching experience. The effects on children of the stresses present in our society—television, video games, drugs, rote learning, family breakdown, peer pressure and others—are such that I find it hard to imagine how a parent can raise balanced, stable, loving, adjusted children without divine guidance. I have been in the homes of many people who have learned the key lessons of successful material plane living, but whose children are in great distress. Spiritual parenting may be the only safe and responsible parenting possible in today's world.

As I witnessed the sensitive and intuitive way in which his mother cared for Lionel as an infant, and as I parented he and Angela in a way that did not conform to much of the parenting I saw around me, many of my old childhood wounds came up to be healed. This is a remarkable discovery: when you commit to a healthy environment for your children, you automatically begin to heal your own childhood. Working on a happy childhood for your children is a sure way to revise your own history.

For me, part of a healthy environment means turning off the TV. We stopped watching with any regularity when Lionel was born, and since then I've lived with little or no TV. As we've stopped pumping pre-packaged images into our minds, our creativity and imagination have blossomed. I've written books, learned to paint, learned ballroom dancing, learned to fly a plane. Cutting off the mass media gives a family many hours in which they can play and explore each other in spontaneous ways. I heartily recommend dropping out in this way. Within a month, you'll wonder how you ever found the time for TV in the first place, as creative and fun activities rush to fill the void left in your time.

Lionel and Angela and I often play board games at night after they've done their homework. One night a week we go Scottish dancing. Sometimes we rent a video, make popcorn, and have a movie party. Or we may go to a movie theater, or a play or performance or event. Sometimes we go to the mall and window shop. Sometimes we do artwork together. Sometimes Lionel and Angela have friends over, but I make sure there's at least one day each week when we're together as a family without other people present, in order to keep our bonding strong.

Selfishly Choosing Joy

Some science fiction stories, and some spiritual teachings, posit the idea of parallel universes. When we reach major points of decision in our lives, so the theory goes, we split, and one reality goes off to experience the results of one decision, while the other diverges with the result of the alternative decision.

I look back at the major decisions in my life, and sometimes wonder what my life would have been like if I'd chosen differently. What would Lionel's life have looked like if he and Angela had not had the kind of spiritual intervention that I've determinedly practiced?

I'm not a strict disciplinarian, but I do decide how I want my family to look, and establish clear and consistent rules for my kids. I don't enforce them absolutely; there's always some give and take. But I've discovered that if I claim the role of the parent clearly and decisively, setting up a consistent structure, my kids are happier and more secure. This promotes joy. And I'm basically selfish: I want a joyful life, and I give consideration to how my life and my family life can be more joyful, then take determined action. I don't leave it to chance!

I've seen many households where the children's whims rule. Two year olds are asked what they would like for dinner, and then the whole family has the same thing, or a parent becomes a short-order chef, cooking individual meals to each person's preferences. Recently, at a park, I saw a little girl continually tripping over her untied shoe laces. Her father said, "Honey, can I tie your shoes?" By giving his daughter a "Yes" or "No" question to answer, this father was handing decision-making over to a child much too young to make that assessment. It is the parents' responsibility to notice and correct unsafe situations like untied shoelaces, not the children's.

While children should be heard and their wants respected, adults are much better equipped, for example, to learn about proper nutrition, and design meals for their families that are healthy and tasty. I find it much harder sometimes to just be the parent, and make the tough decisions, than it would be to give in to children's demands. But I believe it's better in the long run.

Sometimes, maybe once or twice a month, my kids get an ice cream or candy. Angela will ask for an ice cream or candy sometimes several times a day. The day she does get candy in the morning, she'll have forgotten by noon and ask for it again. This puts me in the position of having to say, "No." It's an awkward position, and I see many other parents ducking the issue, and giving in, rather than having the fortitude to judge a child's demand as unreasonable or unhealthy and say, "No." But this is an essential part of being a parent.

Sometimes I joke about this with my kids, when the two of them are arguing about what we should do; I say, "Now let's just pretend for a moment that I'm the parent." This always makes them laugh. Especially since there are days on every vacation when I refuse to be the parent. For a day, I get to be a kid, and refuse to make any decisions. I do this partly for fun, and partly to demonstrate them that "parent" is my role in their lives. And it's simply a role, one I'm taking up for a time and will set down at some later time.

My life seems to have been a difficult one, despite many moments of intense joy. When you commit to living the spiritual life, God believes you, and your psyche believes you. Everything inside you that is unhealed then bursts to the surface. It's a paradox: You pray for Heaven, and out pops Hell! So the years after a spiritual commitment are often filled with turmoil. All the disowned selves within present themselves for healing. Like the knights who sought the Grail, all manner of challenges arise. Staying in Camelot would have been a great deal more comfortable! But the end of the quest is finding yourself, and integrating all the parts of you into a unified, whole person. If you stay true to your soul's quest, no matter how ugly your inside experience is, or how difficult your outside challenges, you gradually heal and clarify those monsters, and take control of your life and your destiny. Love always triumphs.

While my life has had its fair share of sad and difficult moments, a big one came between Lionel's birth and Angela's birth. My wife and I conceived again. We named the baby Montague Augustus. The name we gave the baby was a nod to my family history: Montague was the name of his paternal grandfather, while Augustus was the middle name of George III; my great grandfather five generations back was an illegitimate child of the British king by a woman called Fanny Shelton; during the king's fits of madness he did not demonstrate the sexual restraint that characterized the sane parts of his reign.

It was a difficult pregnancy. My wife's uterus was distended by a large amount of amniotic fluid, much more than normal. We had several sonograms which showed a normal baby boy, but she was kept under close observation by the research hospital at the University of San Francisco until the ninth month.

When the due date for the delivery came around, the baby died in her womb. His heart just stopped beating. She began to hemorrhage massively, and the doctors were concerned we might lose her too.

I prayed with all my might, and I saw angels filling the room. They and I worked on her body using some of the techniques in this book, and the severe internal bleeding suddenly and miraculously stopped, just before she was due to be wheeled into the operating room. She went into labor, with me as her coach, and a few hours later a physically perfect baby boy was born—dead. When she took her fingers and pulled the edges of his mouth upward to see what a smile would have looked like on his sweet face, I hit bottom. Of all the losses in my life, this was perhaps the hardest. I wrote a book about the experience, called *Facing Death, Finding Love*. It is a powerful primer on seeing the face of love through your grief.

When Lionel was seven and Angela was two, their mom and I divorced. Trying to keep a lifeless marriage afloat was literally killing me. My physical body was breaking under the strain.

I then began to slowly figure out—at the age of 40—how to take care of myself. I was good at taking care of a family, I had acquired decent relationship skills, I was great at team work with employees and colleagues and could take care of them, but I had learned very little about how to take care of me. Divorcing was an early step. My inherent joy bobbed to the surface like a cork that had been buried at the bottom of the ocean. My physical body began to bounce back, and I became vibrantly healthy again.

Learning to be happy myself went hand in hand with learning to parent Lionel and Angela well. I pondered on what a happy, emotionally healthy family would look like, and then set out to create one as a single father.

Children and Lovers

The next five years were wonderful for me and my kids. I rediscovered community at a new church, at dances, and with emotionally intimate friends. And through a men's group and men's events, I discovered that male friendships can go very deep. At the same time, my relationships with women were full of both challenge and opportunity. I devoured the opportunity to learn new relationship skills. I treated the challenges that relationships presented as growth opportunities. Yet I discovered that most of the women I met were so deeply wounded, and lost in their wounds, that association with them simply brought that wounding into my life—where it often spilled over to affect my kids. At one point I realized that I had not met a single woman in the previous couple of years who was more fun to be with than my own children, so I gave up dating and just spent time with Lionel and Angela instead!

I also lived with a woman for two years who wanted a child. When she saw the love that I had with my kids, she wanted me to be the father, and we conceived. Then all her deep traumas bubbled to the surface, and she terminated the relationship. Again found myself in a situation from which I had to extricate Lionel and Angela, and, part-time, my new son Alexander.

Not only did I have to deal with a partner's wounds as they surfaced in new relationships. Dealing with my own wounds also engaged me. I tend to embrace growth enthusiastically, no matter how painful it is. So I was grateful whenever a new woman would trigger me, since I then had access to those unresolved issues, and I could work on releasing and healing them. But this took time, and vast amounts of emotional energy. And the women I met seemed to simply be duplicating the wounding experiences of their past relationships, rather than growing past them.

Kids are affected by their parents' dating habits. Kids want their parents to be happy. So they're happy when their parents are happy, and sad when they're not. This exposes them, unfairly I believe, to the emotional ups and downs adults experience in relationships. And when a relationship breaks up, especially if the couple has been living together, the effect on the kids is the loss of a stable household. I imagine excessive use of alcohol or drugs can similarly steal a parent from a child.

The same applies to work. If you're emotionally up when things are going well at work, and down when they're not, your kids can be affected. If you develop habits that support emotional equilibrium, like meditation and inspirational reading, this smoothes out the bumps for both you and your kids.

I've tried to insulate Lionel and Angela from my ups and downs as much as possible, but I've been inconsistent at my success in doing so. My quest for a new mate was my greatest distraction from being fully with my children. If I knew then what I know now, I would have kept my love life on hold for a few years in order to give my kids my full attention.

If you're already in a healthy love relationship, it can contribute to a great family experience with your kids. But be mindful that while your relationship with your children endures till death, the relationship with your current mate may have a much shorter term. And while you may have developed great relationship skills, and formed a high intent, no amount of skill or goodwill is going to work unless the person you're with is taking responsibility for their own inner work and relationship work as well.

There are things you can do, from the outset, to improve your chances. Pick a person who's healthy to start with, who has done intensive work on their old issues. Expect your wounds to come up, take full responsibility for your own experience, don't blame your partner, and heal. Expect their wounds to come up, and be there for your mate if they want to heal too. Read books, take classes, join a support group, hire a therapist or coach, and give yourself every other advantage in the quest for a workable relationship.

Part of male-female relationships is love, magic and chemistry. These things can sustain us in the honeymoon phase of a relationship. But after that, success is largely dependent upon both partners developing good relationship skills. These skills may be as elementary as learning to not interrupt, to keep quiet when your partner is talking. Which technique you embed in your habit set is less important than that you develop mastery of some, any, technique. That way, when you're in the ditch, you have the leverage to pry yourself out. Some that I've found useful are Radical Honesty, (www.radicalhonesty.com), Non-Violent Communication (www.languageofcompassion.com) and Emotional Freedom Technique or EFT (www.emofree.com). These and other resources are listed at the end of this book.

Use and practice the exercises that you learn. At the end of this book is a list of relationship books I've learned from. Memorize your chosen techniques with your mate before you get into trouble, so using them will be an automatic skill when you hit problems. Make agreements to follow certain fight rules, and stick to the agreements that you make.

And if after all this, if the relationship is not working, leave it as quickly and as cleanly as you can.

When Kids Bump Up Against the World

For the first few years of his life, my wife and I were the primary determiners of what Lionel's life looked like. We provided him with a generally loving and safe environment. But gradually, inevitably, he learned about human emotions and behaviors that fall outside the range of love.

Gautama Buddha was raised a prince, groomed to take over his father's kingdom. He grew up entirely within the confines of his father's walled compound, and never saw the suffering of the outside world. Every good thing was provided for him. Only beauty surrounded him. His every need was taken care of.

One day he wandered out of the palace, and came across a sick man, a poor man, and finally a dead man. He had no idea that these states existed. Yet the shock of these opposites led him to begin pondering the great questions of existence, and eventually to enlightenment as he sat beneath the Bodhi tree.

We don't have to abandon our children to the ways of an unconscious world. We don't have to shield them from its realities. We simply need to raise them as caringly as we can, so that they know this mode of being exists, as well as the other.

Lionel first bumped up against the outside world when he was two years old. We were visiting a neighbor—a woman I usually avoided partly because she yelled at her twin toddlers. As the adults were talking, Lionel began to walk down her driveway towards the street. I kept an eye on him, so that I could restrain him if he got too close.

Suddenly the neighbor woman caught sight of him too, and she yelled at him. "Lionel! Don't go in the street!" Lionel was completely overwhelmed. He sat down abruptly, and began to wail. The neighbor sheepishly said, "I guess he's not used to being yelled at." I was sad, yet I knew that I could not insulate Lionel from the ways of the world forever.

When he went to Kindergarten and First Grade, he met kids who were mean to him. He had to get used to the idea that not everybody adored him and would be kind to him, and this idea was not easy for him. It was very difficult for me too. I wondered about home schooling him. Yet I could not play Gautama's father. I reasoned he would need to find out that the world can be challenging at some point during his life, and it might be better to give him a loving household on one hand, so he would know there was another way of being and doing things.

I stayed married for years partly because I didn't want to disrupt Lionel's life by divorce. But eventually things reached the point where I realized that my physical body would soon cease to function if I stayed in the marriage. Leaving it was a matter of literal physical survival.

After I left, and set up my own household, the kids and I began to have a lot more fun. I was liberated from the burden of having to support the relationship, free to be as happy as I chose to be. And that was very, very happy! I could at last create the caring emotional environment I'd always dreamed of. The kids and I had some great years. I bought a gorgeous red Cadillac convertible. The license plate said "Ecstasy." When I picked the kids up from school, we'd put the top down. All three of us would sit in the front seat and we'd yell, "Ecstasy! Ecstasy! Ecstasy!" Seeing each other every day was a return to love.

Even now that Lionel's 15, most mornings I still go into his room to wake him up, hug him in bed, tell him he's a fantastic and inspiring human being and I adore him, and welcome him to the day. Angela gets up in the middle of every night and comes and sleeps half the night with me, as she's done for years.

One effective technique to keep myself mindful of my children, and a very simple one, has been simply tuning in to them when I come home. When Angela talks, I squat down so that I am on her eye level, and listen intently to her. I connect with her exuberant ten-year-old energy, and really inhabit the emotional space she's in. Suddenly I discover that I've for-gotten the cares of my day.

A sure sign for me that I'm off base is when I don't look my kids in the eye when they're addressing me. Another is when I'm listening with half a mind, not really paying attention.

In our family, when a child speaks, everyone listens. I think that chil-dren often yell and act out because no one heeds them when they speak in a normal tone and volume. My kids don't yell, and rarely repeat them-selves. They know that they'll be heard the first time. When Angela speaks, Lionel and I shut up and listen. When I speak, I expect them to do the same. Simply giving children the same respect you would give an adult speaker is one of the most important gifts you can give.

They won't receive the same treatment at school, or see the same behaviors at friends' houses. They may see people ignoring each other and verbally abusing each other.

But they will then have two pictures in their heads, one of an emo-tionally caring household, and one of an emotionally challenged household. When they're setting up their own lives, they can choose. They've seen both modeled, they know what each one looks like, and how they differ.

Although they get little or no TV at home, my kids see it at friends' houses. They've both been through a stage where they wanted to buy everything they saw on TV. They couldn't grasp the concept of ads, that people where trying to convince you of certain beliefs about the value of objects, purely for their own gain. And the materialistic values of our cul-ture seem to seduce my kids as much as others. They judge people by their cars, dress, and how much money they earn. Lionel compares how much he imagines his Christmas present cost with what his sister's cost. He wants to know how much money people earn, and what different jobs pay. He criticizes friends of his who have a little more body fat than he does. He's in horror of ever developing my 40-plus potbelly. The values of our culture are so pervasive, and the countervailing voices so faint, that main-taining children's awareness of the spiritual, the real, takes great effort and awareness on the part of parents. We must speak with a loud, clear, consistent voice for the invisible virtues, and model them in our lives daily.

The bottom line is: You can't protect children from the world. But you can model healthy behaviors at home, so that they know that there are different ways of doing things. And they then have the option of creating a beautiful family when their turn comes along.

On a recent camping vacation, Lionel, Angela and I had lunch at a coffee shop. The establishment was sponsored by three local churches, and Christian sayings, images and paraphernalia were everywhere. Angela called me over to one display, and said, "Daddy, it says something here that's not true." I wondered what could have offended the theological sensibilities of a ten-year-old.

She pointed to a plaque with a photograph of some children her age, inscribed with the words of a song, a song that I remembered well from my own fundamentalist Christian childhood:

> Jesus loves me, this I know
> For the Bible tells me so.
> Little ones to him belong;
> They are weak but he is strong.

"It's not true, Daddy," Angela proclaimed. "Jesus is strong. But we are strong too!" I blessed the Creator in that moment, and in subsequent moments of reflection too, as I realized that despite her goodness and innocence, she lives out of a core conviction that she is strong. As the soul's nature is encouraged to pour out through the child's being, it strengthens all the aspects of mind and heart that are in keeping with its angelic nature. The child can be as strong as God almighty.

When I spend time with kids raised in the mainstream of the cultural paradigm, I realize how different Lionel and Angela are. They listen well. They communicate clearly. They enjoy extended conversations. They are kind to new people; Angela makes a particular point of befriending children who are new to the area. Lionel and Angela notice homeless people on the street, and often give them something. They express love daily. They enjoy physical touch. They often give gifts like massage to other family members without being asked. They are ready to have fun at a moment's notice. They friends they pick at school are the kindest in the class. They are bright and alert, and a joy to be with every single day.

I think they've bought large chunks of the illusion. But is has not taken them over, and I don't believe it ever will. I pray that when their turn comes to choose, they will live in a state of grace.

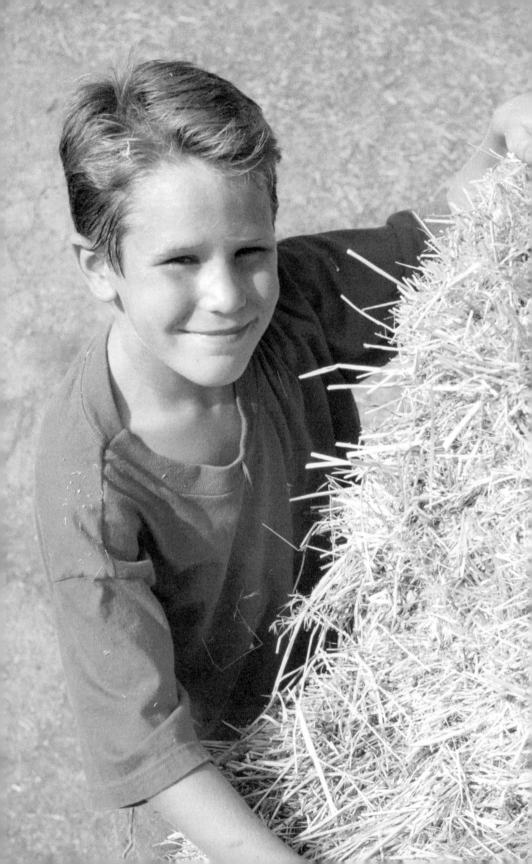

20

Lionel Speaks

What happened in the months and years after Lionel was born? Has his life been marked in any special way? Is he extraordinary in some way as a result of being raised the way he was? Has life been easier for us than it is for other families?

The answer to all these questions is both, "Yes" and, "No."

After he was born, Lionel cried whenever he was awake. Brenda and I couldn't figure out what was bothering him, after exhausting all the obvious possibilities like a dirty diaper, hunger, or cold. Then, after two weeks, I had a sudden insight. I had stopped sharing attunements with him using the methods in this book. Now that he was on the outside of the womb, and I had the visual experience of a baby, the invisible dimensions of his being had receded from my awareness.

I immediately gave him an attunement. His crying stopped right away, and from that moment onward he cried much less. I believe it may have been due to him suddenly finding himself in the same vibrational space as he was so used to in the womb, in the same way that newborns become peaceful and often go to sleep when they're put in cars. They associate car sounds with their long sojourn in the womb. Sharing an attunement told him he was in the same safe space he'd experienced for the previous nine months.

CHAPTER TWENTY

Because children don't have the same fluency with the language as adults do, people often assume that their experiences are less vivid. This is unlikely to be true. Lionel said many things growing up that reminded me that a child's spiritual inner life can be as real, perhaps more real, than any adult's. Here's a sampling of some of the things he said that were precious reminders to me of the presence of God in our lives every day:

Age four: "God loves you so much that he made me out of a loving boy."

Also age four: "When I was asleep, God said in my ear that you're the sweetest boy and you listen to God."

Age five: "The most bestest toy in the world is love."

Age six: "One day I felt God's hands picking me up and holding me. At first I thought it was mom or dad, but it wasn't. I woke up and felt like hands of air were holding me up."

Just before he turned six, he was wrestling with the idea of there being different religions. He said, "Everybody has to worship God. They don't have to worship Jesus, but they do have to worship God."

When Lionel was two, he began to talk about an invisible friend he had called Baybert. Baybert was part of the family for years; Lionel referred to him at least once a month. He told us things that Baybert was doing, and he quickly realized that we could not see or hear Baybert. Baybert seemed to be this big creature, passive and benevolent, that could morph in instant from confidante, to jungle gym, to opposite player in a game. To Lionel, Baybert seemed as matter-of-fact as any corporeal person in his world. Lionel didn't perceive Baybert as anything special; he was apparently able to look from the physical dimension of actual people to the non-dimensional world of discarnate people without any sign of making a transition.

And when Lionel didn't need Baybert any longer, at around age six, Baybert disappeared from Lionel's experience. Brenda and I didn't miss him at first. One day, we realized that Lionel had not talked about Baybert for many months. When we asked where he was, Lionel laughed and told us he wasn't there anymore. Lionel showed no sign of regret; apparently Baybert's memory made him happy but he felt no sense of loss.

Lionel's experience with Baybert made me wonder if some of the invisible friends children talk about are actually guides, or guardian angels. Perhaps they are angels that watch over children in childhood, and stay only while they are needed.

In early 2003 I was working on the revision of this manuscript. Lionel was fourteen years old at that time. I asked Lionel about some of his life experiences. Here, in his own words, is what he said:

"People who don't have a feeling of connection with spirit are sometimes tough inside. A connection with spirit makes me have more concern for other people and life forms; makes me realize that they are beings as well. I see some kids who grew up in situations where their parents were mean to them, and it makes a difference.

"There was a fat boy named Mike in my Cub Scout troop. He was violent, and he would easily fly into a rage. He had no friends. Other kids were scared of him. One day in school he started throwing things around the classroom, and injured a teacher. It took three policemen to hold him to the ground.

"Other kids respond by blowing it off. There's a fourteen-year-old kid in my teen group at church who simply will not open up. Whenever he's asked a question, he says, 'None of your business.' I can see he's scared to open up to other people. I'm very open with other people. Sometimes other kids just don't understand me because I avoid fights, because I'm too gentle. They can't relate to me.

"I remember when my sister was born. I woke up, and there were a whole bunch of people in the house. I got to hold Angela for five minutes, then a midwife took me off to school.

"When I was a baby, all I cared about was playing. 'God' didn't mean much. It was only a word, but one that my parents liked.

"I know that everything is God. Because you see miracles happening all the time. I've got a new baby brother Alexander, and new puppies at the same time. Seeing all these things happen is so profoundly amazing.

"In my teen group at church, everyone is respectful and quiet when we do the meditations. I smile. I feel good, and I think about everyone else in the room. Every insignificant person anywhere has his or her own story. When you look down a street, you realize that each of the people you are seeing has a life as super-complex as your own.

"Sometimes I look at my face in the mirror, and say, 'This is the only me I have.'

"I really like how my dad and my mom have such a good relationship. They're always happy to see each other. Other parents, I see them getting into fights almost every day. But my dad and mom have such a good relationship. The other day they were laughing, he was kidding her about how she never liked him putting photos in albums; she wanted to keep them in shoe boxes instead. They often remember old funny stuff from when they were together. A lot of kids don't have that.

"I feel so connected to men as well as to women. Most other guys I see being scared of being too close to other guys, because that's the way society is. It's so different with me. I can go up to other guys and I have no problem hugging them. They are just other people to me. One of the great things about having a spiritual background is being able to be around other guys without being scared of closeness.

"I've always had one or two people I've especially liked, and could talk to about anything. There was a guy who lived with our family for the first few years after I was born. His name was Jerry. But I never called him that. I called him, 'My Jerry.' He was the first person in my life who I could talk to like that. There's always been someone.

"Many kids have families where the people don't talk and get close. With my Dad, we do a lot of stuff together. Mom I do some stuff together; not as much as I'd like. Mom is basically normal, how other kids are with their moms. Dad and I get closer, because we talk a lot and do a lot of fun stuff together.

"I can't stand hurting other people.

"My friend Jimmy is the worst for this. He's too rough. When he gets in a rough mood, he'll start beating me up. I usually don't fight back because I'm focused on something else I'm doing. I don't like hurting people for real. With Jimmy, if you hurt him, he'll run back at you in a steaming charge, you have to avoid him. He's scary when he's in that mood. I hate that. It's one of the worst things about him. He purposely sends himself into mad rages. He thinks it's fun, but it's scary.

"I got my first experience of people not liking me when I went to kindergarten at Green River Country Day School. There were only two other boys in the class, William and Jake. They were best friends, and they ignored me. That was painful to me. There was more of it at the next school. Last year, one of the girls in my class, Jackie, kicked me so hard she almost broke my rib. Now I know that some people won't like me, so it doesn't matter to me so much any more.

"Sometimes I just sit back and look at what I have and think, 'Gee, I'm lucky.' My friend Jimmy always wants more. He's never happy just with what he has. You never see him look at something he owns and say, 'Isn't this great!' He wants the next best thing.

"My dad told me about this culture where a family puts all their possessions in a heap every few years and burns the lot. The people who burn the biggest pile are thought to be the richest families. That's awesomely cool, when you don't have to feel any thing is so precious that you can't live without it."

Further Reading

RELATIONSHIP BOOKS

Don't Be Nice, Be Real, by Kelly Bryson, MFT. (Elite, 2005).

Keeping the Love You Find, by Harville Hendrix, Ph.D. (Pocket, 1993).

Practicing Radical Honesty, by Brad Blanton, Ph.D., (Sparrowhawk, 2000).

A General Theory of Love, by Fari Amini, Richard Lannon, and Lewis Thomas, M.D. (Vintage, 2001).

The New Couple, by Maurice Taylor and Seana McGee. (HarperCollins, 2000).

Be Loved For Who You Really Are, by Judith Sherven and James Sniechowski. (Renaissance, 2001).

Conscious Loving, by Gay and Kathlyn Hendricks. (Bantam, 1992).

How Loving Couples Fight, by James Creighton. (Aslan, 1998).

The Eight Essential Traits of Couples Who Thrive, by Susan Page, Ph.D. (DTP, 1997).

Discovering Sexuality that will Satisfy You Both, by Anne Hastings, Ph.D. (Printed Voice, 1993).

The Illuminated Chakras, a stunning DVD journey through the chakras by Anodea Judith, Ph.D. (www.sacredcenters.com).

The Emotional Freedom Technique EFT Video Course, by Gary Craig. EFT is a remarkable technique that can heal many emotional and physical ailments permanently in just a few minutes. (www.emofree.com).

PARENTING BOOKS

Giving the Love that Heals, by Harville Hendrix, Ph.D. and Helen Hunt, M.A. (Pocket, 1997).

Radical Parenting, by Brad Blanton, Ph.D. (Sparrowhawk, 2002).

Parenting as a Spiritual Journey, by Nancy Fuchs (Jewish Lights, 1998).

The Continuum Concept, by Jean Liedloff (Perseus, 1986).

The Natural Child, by Jan Hunt & Peggy O'Mara (New Society, 2001).

The Joyful Child, by Peggy Jenkins, Ph.D. (Aslan, 1996).

Journey of Awakening, by Ram Dass. (Bantam, 1990).

The Seven Spiritual Laws for Parents, by Deepak Chopra. (Harmony, 1997).

WEB SITES

This book's web site..www. Communing.com

Alliance for Transforming the Lives of Children...........www.aTLC.org

Jeannine Parvati Baker ....www.BirthKeeper.com

Radical Honesty ....www.RadicalHonesty.com

Non Violent Communication ....www.LanguageOfCompassion.com

Anodea Judith's Chakra Site ....www.SacredCenters.com

Emotional Freedom Technique ....www.EmoFree.com

Neale Donald Walsch....................................www.HumanitysTeam.com

Gay and Kathlyn Hendricks ....www.Hendricks.com

The Emissaries ....www.Emissaries.org

Byron Katie...www.TheWork.org

Harville Hendrix..www.Imagotherapy.com

OTHER BOOKS BY THE AUTHOR

The meditations from *Communing With the Spirit of Your Unborn Child* are available in a downloadable audio version from www.Communing.com for $15.

The Heart of Healing. An anthology including chapters by Andrew Weil, Deepak Chopra, Dean Ornish, Joan Borysenko, Bernie Siegel, Jeanne Achterberg and others, edited by Dawson Church. (Elite Books, 2004). Hardback, $25.

Facing Death, Finding Love: The Healing Power of Grief and Loss in One Family's Life. (Aslan, 1994). Softcover, $10.95.

Healing Our Planet, Healing Our Selves. An anthology including chapters by Huston Smith, The Dalai Lama, Deepak Chopra, Neale Donald Walsch, Gay Hendricks, Helen Caldicott, Mary Catherine Bateson, Andrew Harvey, and many others, edited by Dawson Church (Elite Books, 2005). Hardback, $25

To order a book by the author, send a check for the amount plus $3 shipping to the address on the author's web site at www.Communing.com.

PROCLAMATION FOR TRANSFORMING THE LIVES OF CHILDREN

The following proclamation for transforming the lives of children comes off the web site of The Alliance for Transforming the Lives of Children, (www.aTLC.org, © 2001), and is a ringing statement of the ideals that I believe hold the potential of transforming child-raising in this century.

WE ENVISION A WORLD WHERE

- Every child is wanted, welcomed, loved, and valued;
- Every family is prepared for and supported in practicing the art and science of nurturing children;
- Adults respect children and honor childhood;
- Children joyfully participate in the life of family and community; and
- Dynamic, resilient, life-honoring cultures flourish.

WE WILL CREATE THIS WORLD BY

- Recognizing that in nature's design there are biological imperatives (ranging from mere physical survival—food, water, air, and shelter— to those that foster optimal human development) that must be fulfilled to support optimal human development;
- Identifying the evidence-linked principles that arise from these imperatives; and
- Acting on these principles that are essential for transforming the lives of children.

CHILDREN ARE IN CRISIS

28%: Pregnant women subjected to physical or emotional violence. (Department of Women's Health, World Health Organization.)

0%: Infant male circumcisions that are medically indicated or beneficial. (American Medical Association, Council on Scientific Affairs.)

85.5%: American infants denied the benefits of breastfeeding for the one-year minimum recommended by the American Academy of Pediatrics. (Ross Laboratory's Annual Mothers' Survey, 1998.)

25%: Children documented to have been physically struck by age 6 mo. (*Bearing Witness: Violence and Collective Responsibility,* Hayworth Press, S.L. Bloom and M. Richert.)

92%: Number of infant and toddler facilities that fail to meet minimum standards. (University of Colorado, Denver, Economics Department: Cost, quality, and Child outcomes study team.)

40%: Children living apart from biological father. (US Bureau of the Census, *Current Population Reports,* 1997.)

20%: Children ages 6-12 who have not had a 10-minute conversation with a parent in a month. (Children's Defense Fund.)

16,000: Number of murders witnessed on TV and computer games by the average child before reaching school age. (American Medical Association. *Physician Guide to Media Violence,* 1996.)

200%: Increase in suicide, ages 5-14 (5th leading cause of death) since 1979. (US National Center for Health Statistics, CDC, July 2001.)

9 million: US children under 18 estimated suffering from a psychiatric disorder that compromises their ability to function. (National Institute of Mental Health)

1.6 million: Number of arrests of children under 18 in US per year. (US Department of Justice)

5 million: US pre-schoolers living below the poverty line. (US Bureau of the Census, *Current Population Reports,* 1997.)

"Never before has one generation of American children been less healthy, less cared for, or less prepared for life than their parents were at the same age." (National Association of State Boards of Education, 1990.)

"Never before has there been such a wealth of information on keeping children healthy, caring for them, and preparing them for life." (The Alliance for Transforming the Lives of Children, 2001.)

PRINCIPLES FOR TRANSFORMING THE LIVES OF CHILDREN

aTLC's philosophy: Children are innately good, cooperative, and whole in spirit. Parents do the best they can at any given moment, within their present situation and life circumstances. Agreement on a set of guiding principles by all family members promotes enjoyable, confident parenting and provides children with a consistent, supportive environment.

aTLC offers the following evidence-linked Principles for promoting optimal human development. Our deep concern for children and parents is woven into each Principle. We invite you to ponder these Principles that we hope will motivate and inspire you. We encourage you to recognize and follow your intuitive knowledge and instincts. Our intent is to help you co-create with children a life that is practical, harmonious, and joyful.

1.   All children are born with inherent physical, emotional, intellectual, and spiritual needs that, when met, foster optimal human development.

Emotional needs for unconditional love, touch, and attention are as valid as physical needs. Responding to crying rather than leaving children alone to "cry it out" shows them that their needs are acknowledged and deepens their basic trust.

2.   Every child needs to be securely bonded with at least one other person—optimally the mother.

The infant-mother bond is primary and lays the foundation for all future relationships.

Securing and maintaining a strong bond is the foundation of a parent's effectiveness and the key to a child's optimal development.

3.   All children are by nature social beings, born with the drive to play, learn, cooperate with others, and contribute to their world.

Children are more able to reach their full potential when treated with respect within a loving environment that meets their emotional and physical needs, and encourages and supports innate curiosity and spontaneous learning.

Flexibility, clear thinking, age-appropriate problem solving, and intuition are optimized in a child-led learning environment that offers clear, consistent boundaries along with creative, cooperative activities, interaction with nature, unstructured play, and time to simply be.

4. Each child carries within a unique pattern of development designed to unfold in accordance with the child's own rhythm and pace. Every child deserves trust and respect for her or his own emerging learning styles and abilities. Parents who perceive their child's pattern of development are better able to nurture their child in harmony with this pattern.

5. Young children communicate their needs through behavior that is strongly influenced by innate temperament, early experiences, the behavior modeled by others, and current circumstances. Children naturally imitate those around them. When adults discover what a child's behavior is actually communicating, they are better able to respond to the need rather than react to the behavior.

6. The ability of parents and caregivers to nurture children is strongly influenced by their own birth, childhood, and life experiences.

The more adults understand and compensate for their own unmet physical and emotional childhood needs, the better able they are to meet the needs of children in their care.

Once they are better informed, parents who lacked adequate information, resources, or support during the earlier stages of their children's development can strive to compensate for unmet needs.

7. Children depend upon their parents and caregivers to keep them safe and to protect them from emotional and physical neglect, violence, sexual abuse, and other toxic conditions. Violence, such as infant circumcision, spanking, shaming, and emotional abuse weakens or impairs children's sense of wholeness, trust, and security.

Toxic influences that damage children's brains and nervous systems include over-stimulation from video games, computers, and television, as well as environmental contaminants and behavior-modifying drugs.

8. A child who is nurtured in the womb of a healthy, loving, and tranquil mother receives the best possible start in life.

The unborn child is a sensitive being who is aware of, and responsive to, the mother's feelings and experience.

A growing life is strongly influenced by the mother's physical, mental, and emotional wellbeing, as well as the quality of support she receives throughout pregnancy.

9. A natural birth affords significant benefits to mother and baby; therefore, both the potential benefits and risks of any intervention warrant careful consideration.

A natural birth is more likely to occur in an environment based on the midwifery model of care, with physical and emotional support, nourishment, freedom of movement, and individualized attention.

The possible benefits of any contemplated test, procedure, drug, or surgery must be weighed against the immediate and long-term risks, according to current scientific evidence.

10. Breastfeeding, continual physical contact, and being carried on the body are necessary for optimal brain and immune system development, and promote the long-term health of the baby and mother.

Spontaneous breastfeeding for a minimum of two years supports optimal bonding, immunity, and nutrition.

Carrying infants in-arms or wearing them in slings throughout the day provides the near-constant movement that optimizes brain development as well as the touch, safety, and comfort essential to secure bonding.

11. A father's consistent, meaningful, and loving presence in a child's life is significant to the child, father, mother, and the wellbeing of the family.

The father's role may begin with preparation for conception and continues with the physical and emotional protection and support of the mother, baby, and mother-child bond.

In the absence of the biological father, a bonded, ongoing relationship with a loving male caregiver is optimal for every child.

12. Parents create a strong foundation for family life when they consciously conceive, foster, or adopt a child, and are committed to understand and meet the child's needs.

Parents welcome children best when they consciously prepare their own bodies, minds, and spirits for pregnancy and birth, and think of conception as a deep commitment between themselves and the baby.

Even when pregnancy is unplanned, both parents can create a healthy, nurturing environment for their child.

13. Single parents have a special need for a strong emotional and financial support system to effectively nurture their children.

Respecting and supporting a child's healthy relationship with each parent is essential to the child's self-confidence and self-value.

A support system that includes healthy-functioning adults of both genders and multiple generations provides balanced nurturing and role modeling.

14. Political, economic, and social structures either enhance or diminish parents' opportunities to nurture and sustain a secure bond with their children. Support from the immediate community and society at large is crucial if parents are to maintain a secure bond with their children in a nuclear family structure.

Society benefits and families thrive when health care and socio-political structures support all families in preparing for optimal gestation, birth, and parenting.

15. When children live in socially responsive families and communities, they receive a foundation for becoming socially responsible themselves. Children learn to respect and respond to the needs of others when they are seen and heard, and their opinions and needs are recognized, respected, and met.

Engaging children in age-appropriate, creative, and compassionate problem solving and decision-making within the family and the community fosters their becoming responsible members of a society.

16. Effective parenting is an art that can be learned.

Information about children's developmental stages, temperament, and individuality helps parents make informed decisions and serve as advocates of the child's wellbeing. Ready access to evidence-linked information about optimal human development is vital for societies that have departed from nature's biological imperatives.

By implementing these Principles through Actions such as those suggested in the aTLC Blueprint, societies can transform themselves into dynamic, life-honoring cultures where children are loved, protected, respected, valued, and encouraged to joyfully participate in the vital life of family and community.